The
Perimenopause
JOURNAL

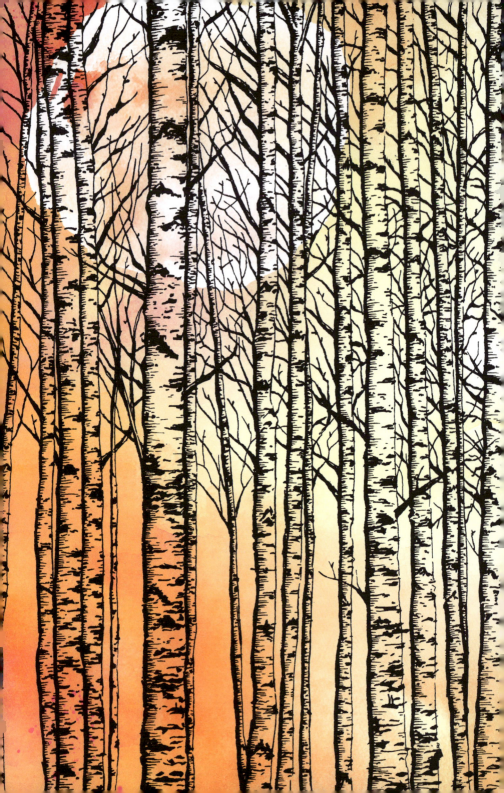

The
Perimenopause
JOURNAL

KATE CODRINGTON

Unlock your power
Own your wellbeing
Find your path

DAVID & CHARLES

www.davidandcharles.com

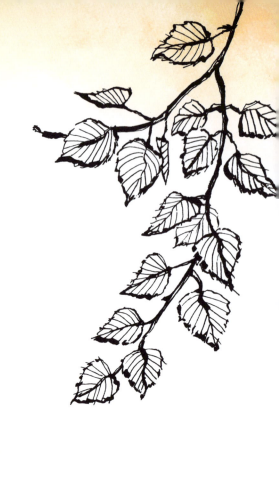
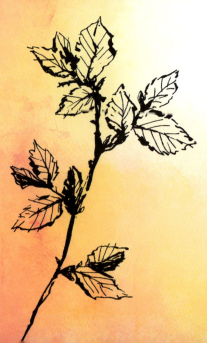

Contents

Charting Your Path to Second Spring

Perimenopause is not a hormone deficiency, it's the time before your last period, a normal life stage and transition to a more liberating time of life. Perimenopause need not be a crisis, but lots of people talk up a fearful narrative that creates stress and confusion, which will make symptoms worse. Lots of people can make lots of money by suggesting that your body is failing and falling apart. Perimenopause is a time of growth that is asking you to love yourself more. But there's not much money to be made in us blossoming on our own terms. So what's going on?

It is clear that we have not been living in a sustainable way: our exhaustion, the planet's crisis, the lack of care for our wellbeing, especially in perimenopause, the endless misogyny and the way we fear ageing show us clearly that we are working out of step with the natural rhythm of life. It's not us malfunctioning here, it's the system that's at fault. We know this in our bones, but nevertheless we resist and fight against the natural ebb and flow, and continue to suffer.

Living with the seasons, known as cyclical living or cyclical awareness, brings us into a more caring relationship with the earth and with ourselves. The seasons also appear as 'inner seasons' through our reproductive lives in the menstrual and moon cycles. We become increasingly expansive through our inner Springs and Summers, and more reflective and inward-looking through our inner Autumns and Winters. Since your first period you've been in an expansive Spring and Summer phase, and the more reflective Autumn and Winter of your perimenopause has likely come as a shock because we were told the expansion was limitless: we should keep on giving and multi-tasking forever. But there has to be a time of reflection, releasing and rest before we can emerge into postmenopause, also known as your Second Spring, with the energy to start a fresh cycle. To put it simply, if you want to emerge into a badass Second Spring, you'll probably need to drop some less helpful habits and beliefs.

These same inner seasons are present in the menstrual cycle, and paying attention to what trips you up and what supports you in your premenstrual phase will show you how to care for yourself in perimenopause. Your cycle has been preparing you

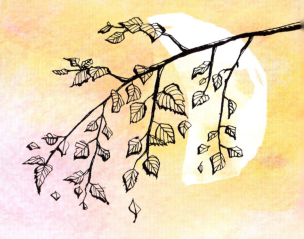

for perimenopause all this time. How about that?! By following this innate ebb and flow, we can open the way to better health and also to a more creative and soulful, happier life. The inner seasons were developed by menstrual educators Red School, whom I've been lucky enough to work with – this journal and my first book *Second Spring* are largely based on what I've learned from them.

Perimenopause is actually much more than just the time before periods stop. It is a time of psychological exploration, when we examine where we've come to, what we had to do to get here, what to let go of and how we'd like to be postmenopause. It is a time when we are preparing for the second cycle of our lives, and bringing a seasonal lens is absolute gold as we ponder how to live to the max, on our own terms and without burning out, so we can thrive in the second half of our lives.

This journal walks you step by step through how to recognise the seasons within you and most importantly, how to care for yourself. By tracking your progress with the journal and using yoga nidra meditations, you can surf the wave of change through perimenopause as a process of deepening self-love and awareness. Unusually for a book about perimenopause, you won't find any lists of symptoms here. Instead there's a warm invitation to discover how it feels to be you.

You have been challenging norms all your life, getting curious about what's going on behind the green curtain, trying to figure out how to connect more deeply with yourself and the planet, and still enjoy a cheeky cocktail before heading home. If you go to yoga, but cringe at the chanting, or close your mindfulness class with a glass of prosecco and still yearn for a deeper connection with yourself, you're in the right place. I've got you!

My intention for this journal is that it becomes a safe space, away from the misogyny and fear that surround perimenopause, to support you to find connection and trust as you navigate towards the best half of your life.

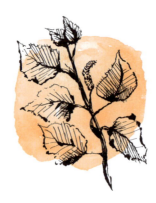

About me

Who am I to be asserting this liberating weirdness? Let's start with the personal.
I'm postmenopausal and can honestly say that I am happier now than I have
ever been. After years of feeling not good enough and mysteriously wonky, I
have stopped wasting energy worrying about what other people think and can
now pursue what makes me happy. I've stopped feeling glum about the way
I look and instead, I celebrate what my strong, beautiful, older body can do.
After years of dithering I make decisions based on my gut feelings and intuition.
And finally, finally, I find I can care for myself with increasing compassion,
and when things go wrong, I can set myself gently back on my bicycle and
wobble off again. I am not special or unusual. Not at all. I see this increasing
freedom from 'shoulds' and 'oughts' in all my clients, in the groups I facilitate
and in my community of folk who are navigating perimenopause. There is,
just under our noses, a movement that liberates us from being 'not enough',
which naturally occurs through perimenopause and menopause, and instead
offers us a vibrant and creative postmenopausal life in which we can know,
finally, that we were enough all the time. Professionally I have been a therapist
for more than 30 years and have witnessed thousands of people finding
more self-acceptance, creativity and joy from connecting with the seasons
of the body. I am your chief validation officer and this journal will validate the
importance of your needs and feelings – and that you already know how to
care for yourself – you just need gentle guidance and awareness to find them.

Benefits of tracking

The benefits of tracking are endless, but when it's hard to remember what you went into a room for, let alone when you started those supplements, writing things down is essential. The suggestions I'm offering are based on what's been helpful for my clients through their transitions, but you may have other issues to track over the months. Here's how tracking can help you:

- Identifying what inner season you're in is an easy route to self-care.

- The more you track your self-care, the more powerful and accessible your toolkit will become.

- Noting your emotions validates your experience, reduces judgement and helps you claim more of your range of being.

- Tracking your energy levels can help you recognise your boundaries and how you might need replenishment.

- Setting intentions for the lunar or menstrual month helps you align yourself with your values and not get so side-tracked.

- Writing down when you started taking medication or supplements will help you see how much they're helping.

- It also provides solid data for any health professionals that are supporting you.

- Noting changes in diet, both positive and negative, will help you see how they have affected you over time.

- Celebrations. I like to celebrate every win I can. Even getting out of bed counts as a triumph sometimes.

- Gratitude has been shown to make us happier. Simple. Quick. Effective. Why wouldn't you?

Given that period tracking apps can be a privacy nightmare, paper is the way forward, offering a simple, embodied, mindful practice available to you every day.

The Seasons

Before we get into detail, here's a quick low-down on the seasons:

Spring and Summer
Increasingly engaging with the world

Autumn and Winter
Increasingly engaging with our inner selves

Take a look at the illustration of the seasonal cycle here. Note that you've been rolling through these four phases since your periods began, and they will continue as you move into perimenopause and beyond. What season are you in right now? If you're full of beans and love that beautiful face in the mirror, you're probably in Summer. Prickly, saying no, hot on boundaries, clearing your cupboards or standing your ground? That's Autumn. Dreamy, longing to nap, low energy and craving a duvet day? Winter calling! Full of wonder and possibilities, with the legs of Bambi and eyes like dinner plates? That's Spring for you.

All seasons can show up in your days, regardless of your cycle: just noticing where you're at right now is all you need to do.

Summer

Ovulation

20s-30s

healthy ego
effectiveness
productivity

Autumn

Premenstrual phase
Perimenopause

discernment
truth telling
empowerment

BLOSSOM

FRUIT

INCREASING EXPANSION
capacity + outward focus

INCREASING CONTRACTION
sensitivity + inward focus

GROW

SEED

Spring

Post-menstruation
Postmenopause & teens

wonder
playfulness
possibilities

Winter

Menstruation
Menopause

self-acceptance
spirituality
healing

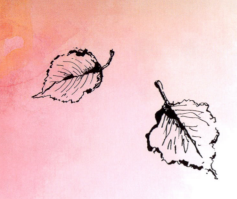

The inner seasons show up in the four phases of the menstrual cycle and are also present in the longer arc of our lives, giving us an anchor in times of uncertainty, like perimenopause and the premenstrual phase, both autumnal seasons. The two halves of the cycle create a natural balance between activity and rest, service to others and service to ourselves. Each season has challenges and gifts that are generalised across many people's experience, but you will discover your own flavour and particular take on things as you track your inner seasons. You'll notice different seasons through your day, as well as seasons influenced more by your menstrual cycle, the moon and your time of life. Confusing? Not at all! All you need do is notice where you're at now and care for that. Nothing more.

Part of the exhaustion we're feeling is because we are resisting the season we're in: we push through till we're on our knees. The shame and sense of failure we feel from not being bright and shiny all the time can be crippling, as we stifle our needs and mask our inner selves to keep up with our perceived 'normal'. By accepting the season we are in and giving ourselves pockets of appropriate care, we can slow our pace and protect ourselves when needed, and also allow for enthusiastic multi-tasking when that becomes possible again.

The seasons have your back, just lean in and let yourself be held.

Menstrual seasons

For many people, perimenopause first makes an appearance in the second half of the menstrual cycle – in the premenstrual phase and period – often announcing herself with the screaming heebie-jeebies and trailing chaos in her wake. But even if you don't currently have a menstrual cycle, it's still interesting to reflect back on your past experience of the cyclical seasons as this can inform your present Autumns.

Why on earth would you be interested in becoming aware of your cycle, just at the point when you're saying farewell? Giving attention to your departing cycle can deliver multiple rewards. For example, your premenstrual phase gives you loads of insight into how to manage yourself through perimenopause: what triggers you, what might be causing this and what you can do to ease the discomfort. Grief is also part of the perimenopausal, autumnal picture, and acknowledging what you are letting go of is part of the grief process. Whatever your relationship to your cycle has been through your life, saying goodbye to it is a rite of passage and it's hard to get closure when you haven't fully greeted your cycle while it was present. Noticing the nuance of your feelings and the length and qualities of your menstrual flow will also help you see where you are in your menopause process, giving a sense of anchoring into the wider flow of your life. In the next part of this book you'll find the low-down on the archetypal menstrual seasons and how to care for them, but first let me introduce you to yoga nidra.

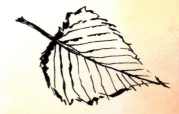

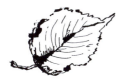

Introducing yoga nidra

If these ideas about inner seasons are new to you, you're likely to have lots of questions, and be trying to figure it all out and understand how it fits in with your lived experience. But this is not something you can master with intellect alone. Cyclical awareness needs a combination of curiosity, as well as body and emotional awareness that builds over time. There is however a handy short-cut in the form of gentle yoga nidra meditations, which I refer to in the seasonal guides that follow.

Yoga nidra are guided meditations that lead you gently into a relaxed, slightly altered state of consciousness between sleeping and waking that can be close to bliss. You may well have received one already, in the relaxation session at the end of a yoga class. Probably you'll fall asleep when you do nidra, but that's fine too, it's an adaptive practice and even while you're asleep your unconscious will still be open to the healing.

You are fully entitled to rest. In preparation for nidra meditation, I warmly invite you to put your life to one side for 20 minutes, and settle into your favourite spot, whether it's your bed, sofa or armchair. Gather cushions, a blanket and your favourite socks to nestle in for some seriously luxe rest.

The nidra will integrate your understanding of each inner season effortlessly with peace, grounding, and access to intuition and spirituality.

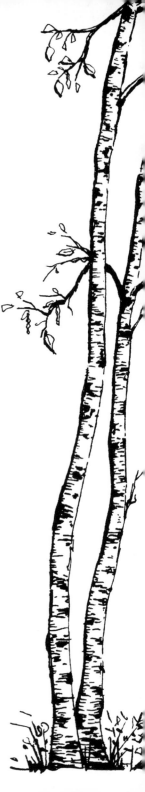

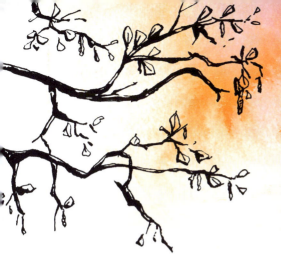

Yoga nidra ticks so many boxes: you get to rest, it requires no skill or experience, you are encouraged to respond with kindness to your body and mind, and meanwhile, without any effort at all, your subconscious can learn and integrate new information.

Now let's turn to the path that winds through our seasonal experience of our monthly cycles, beginning with Winter...

Audio guides for meditation

For each season I have created a yoga nidra that not only gives you a precious pocket of rest, but also integrates the gifts and qualities of each season without any effort or prior experience on your part. You don't have to be an ace meditator or do anything at all to be able to enjoy them.

I have also recorded a guided meditation that's designed to support you as you set some intentions to help you navigate each month in the journal section of this book.

To access any of the audio guides, just scan the QR code using your smartphone, and tap on the link that it brings up.

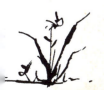

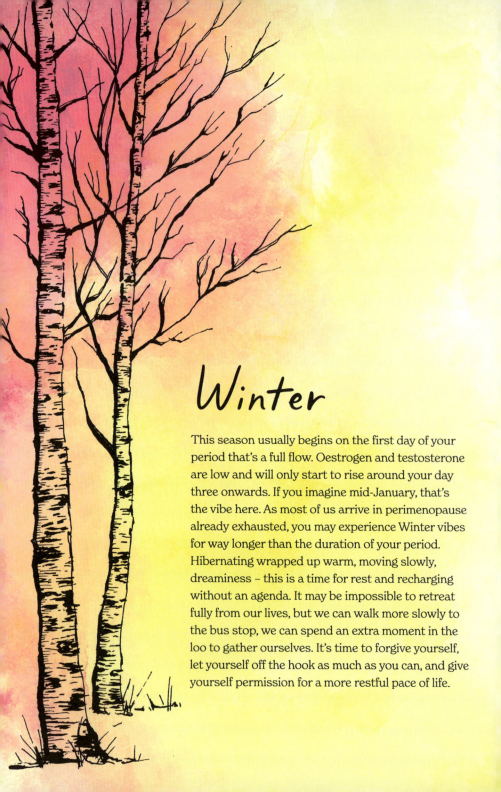

Winter

This season usually begins on the first day of your period that's a full flow. Oestrogen and testosterone are low and will only start to rise around your day three onwards. If you imagine mid-January, that's the vibe here. As most of us arrive in perimenopause already exhausted, you may experience Winter vibes for way longer than the duration of your period. Hibernating wrapped up warm, moving slowly, dreaminess – this is a time for rest and recharging without an agenda. It may be impossible to retreat fully from our lives, but we can walk more slowly to the bus stop, we can spend an extra moment in the loo to gather ourselves. It's time to forgive yourself, let yourself off the hook as much as you can, and give yourself permission for a more restful pace of life.

WINTER SELF-CARE

Slowing down

Put your phone down, walk more slowly, do only what is essential, make space between commitments.

Resting

Find something restful that eases your mind and make it a non-negotiable part of your Winter days. If you haven't already, try a yoga nidra meditation.

Receiving

It's time to give yourself extra nourishment from food that you cooked earlier in your cycle, receive help and support from others and let yourself be held, where that's available to you.

Pottering

An excellent way of giving your whole system a break, and getting out of your own way so the wisdom of the cycle can hold you.

Use your Summer energies to educate your loved ones about the seasons and to set up help for your inner Winters.

REST

Most of us arrive at perimenopause bloody exhausted, with no reserves available for the work of transformation. No wonder it's hard. In this perimenopausal state our primary self-care is to rest, so that we can have space to see what needs releasing, and so that over time we can refill our boots and claw back our resources.

Resting isn't necessarily lying down: one person's rest is another person's torture and lying down can be too agitating for some people. Even slowing down can be a challenge after speeding along for four decades, so it's important to find something restful you can regularly engage in. When something is restful for you, your breath will slow and deepen, your heart-rate slow down, your shoulders soften and your thoughts become more spacious. It's anti-inflammatory too! It might be colouring, walking, gardening, my beloved yoga nidra – hell it can even be tidying or cleaning. It's time to lift the lid on rest: how to do it, and what to do, even when life continues to break over your head in a tsunami of demands.

Ask yourself

What tends to get in the way of you resting? Try journalling on the prompt: 'If I rested as much as I need to then....'. The more specific you can be, the better.

Listen to the phrases and voices that come up in your response. How can you address these? For example, if your inner voice tells you you're lazy if you rest more, and that other people can hold it together so you should too, can you access a more compassionate voice, like a best friend or someone whose self-care you admire, and wonder how they might respond?

What is restful for you?

How can you commit to more of that in your life?

Top tip

Pottering is a much underrated art – moving around your space without aims or goals, gently enjoying domestic safety. It has the advantage of looking like a purposeful task contributing to humanity, when in fact you are drifting about.

SMALL PLEASURES

Pleasure has an astonishing range of physiological and psychological benefits. It improves happiness, heart health, immunity, sexual response, hormone balance, bone health and relationships too. It doesn't have to be complicated. By engaging the senses, looking at beautiful things, laughing, hugging, self-touch, dancing, these regular, small doses of pleasure gently bring us back to life, almost like the magic perimenopause pill we dream of.

But often it's hard to allow ourselves enough pleasure. We feel it's too indulgent or superficial or a waste of time, and instead of claiming a little pleasure-time every day, we bundle up massive expectations on a rare spa day or night out. It's not enough. We need regular doses of 'vitamin P' to make it through.

A menopause symptom that is surprisingly common, yet seldom mentioned, is joylessness. Akin to depression, it can hang around for years and make living feel pointless and even bring suicide ideation. When our expression is blocked, for example by a controlling partner, unwelcome caring duties, financial hardship or disability, joylessness can result. Often we are powerless to change our circumstances, but we can nudge our experience into more flow with pleasure.

Ask yourself

What were the prevailing beliefs about pleasure when you were growing up?

How are these beliefs operating in your life now?

Do they serve you?

What kinds of pleasure are most accessible for you? Do you love music? Is it wonderful food, beautiful perfume or a tender touch that turns you on? Does this work best alone, with a special person or in a group? List the kind of things you want more of.

How can you bring pockets of pleasure into your daily life now?

Winter self-care at a glance

It's time to refill your cup with nourishment: good food, good movement, good rest, nature and time.

WINTER CHALLENGES

Constantly ignoring the need for refilling your cup in Winter, and pushing through, will contribute to burnout and more troubling perimenopause symptoms. We can contract in our Winters, with an existential fear they might never end, that we're are stuck here and this season will never, ever shift. It's as though we are facing our mortality, and here, each time we meet our Winter, we do indeed have the opportunity to do that. If you look at the opposite side of the cycle, in high Summer, are you tempted to feel that we've finally got life sorted and Summer will never end? Winter is the necessary polar opposite.

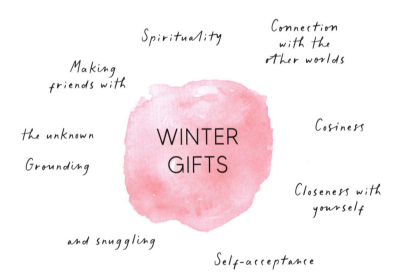

Spirituality

Connection with the other worlds

Making friends with

the unknown

Grounding

WINTER GIFTS

Cosiness

Closeness with yourself

and snuggling

Self-acceptance

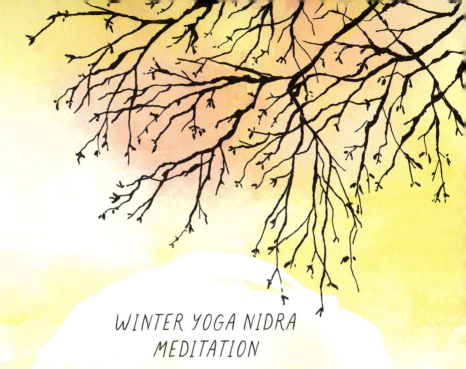

WINTER YOGA NIDRA MEDITATION

At this natural time to rest and go inwards, you may find a Winter-related nidra particularly useful if you're burnt out, exhausted, menstruating or grieving. Taking shelter in the dreamy nidra landscape will help you rest and resource yourself for the hibernation period, as you invite peace into all parts of the body. What a relief from fighting all the flipping time! A sensory exploration of a Winter landscape can help you integrate the Winter qualities of spirituality, receiving, vision, trust and self-compassion. You can reengage with the world with the courage to go at your own pace.

To listen to the yoga nidra, simply scan this QR code on your smartphone and choose from the audio files on offer.

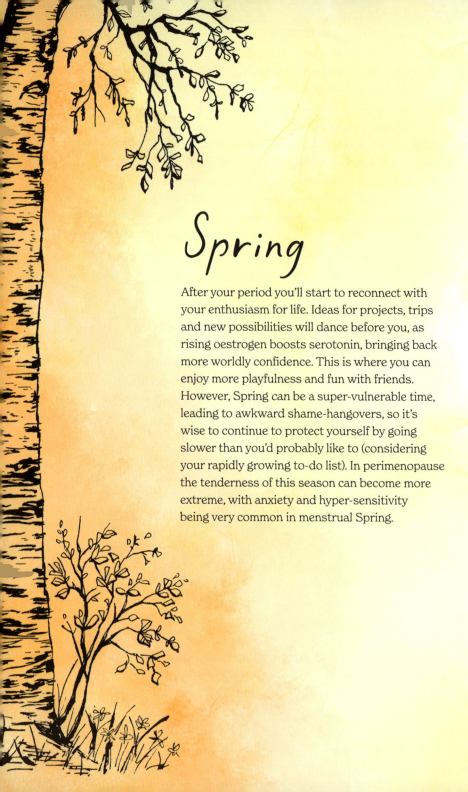

Spring

After your period you'll start to reconnect with your enthusiasm for life. Ideas for projects, trips and new possibilities will dance before you, as rising oestrogen boosts serotonin, bringing back more worldly confidence. This is where you can enjoy more playfulness and fun with friends. However, Spring can be a super-vulnerable time, leading to awkward shame-hangovers, so it's wise to continue to protect yourself by going slower than you'd probably like to (considering your rapidly growing to-do list). In perimenopause the tenderness of this season can become more extreme, with anxiety and hyper-sensitivity being very common in menstrual Spring.

SPRING SELF-CARE

Playing

Drop the goals and do
something 'just because'. Play
creates joy, intimacy, creativity,
improved neural connections
and emotional resilience.

Protection

Be careful of who and
what you let near you.
Avoid 'joy vampires', bullies
and competitive types.

Soothing your nervous system

Get into your version of
nature, surrounding yourself
with reassuring smells, self-
touch and grounding.

Have a notebook dedicated to Spring ideas
and possibilities so you can catch them before
they get in the hands of your inner critic.

ON MOVEMENT

Movement in the body supports movement in the whole system: mood, vitality, hormonal health, digestion, the lot, particularly when it's of the pleasurable variety. A body in movement literally cannot stay the same. Think of a class of nursery school kids – none of them stay still for more than a second; their natural life force demands to be expressed at all times. At the other end of life, in so-called 'Blue Zones' – the places that have the highest number of centenarians – the inhabitants are found to be naturally inclined to move more, and this is identified as part of the secret of a long and healthy life.

However, perimenopause can bring on a kind of frozen state where we are immobilised by exhaustion, fear, overwhelm or all three together. As it progresses it contributes to the feeling that this awfulness will never end, we are stuck here for good and rather than being in transition, we've already hit crone-dom and might as well give up. We're on our knees. Any movement – apart from reaching for the biscuits – seems beyond our capabilities. This becomes a catch-22: the more static we are in our bodies, the more stuck our minds become and it can feel as if there's no way out.

How can we move out of 'stuckness' when we are exhausted?

Try this

Bringing your attention to your body as it is now, scan through from crown to toes, and note: where do you notice sensation and where is there less or no sensation? Just greet all the sensation and no-sensation parts with curiosity and warmth – there are no judgements here.

Taking one part with sensation, with a playful attitude, see how it would like to move; just follow any impulse and see what happens for a moment or two. All are welcome, from giant moves to invisible wiggles. If you don't detect any impulse, make it up, see what happens. Then, coming back to stillness, scan through again from crown to toe and notice any changes.

Taking one part with less or no sensation, with a playful attitude, explore how this body part can move. Follow any impulse and see what happens for a moment or two. All are welcome, from huge moves to invisibly tiny wiggles. Again, if you don't detect any impulse, make it up and see what happens. Then, once more coming back to stillness, scan through from crown to toe and notice any changes.

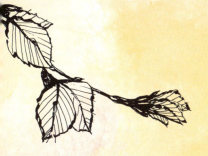

Ask yourself

In your current and past life, what kind of movement was fun and pleasurable? Dancing around? Stomping up a hill? Swinging, shaking, spinning around in the playground? Make a list of pleasurable moves.

How can you build more pleasurable movement breaks into your days?

Top tips

Exercise 'snacks' of 10 minutes are shown to have as much benefit as longer sessions. Here are some ideas to build more movement into your day even when you're exhausted.

- Go outside for a walk, or stretch in the morning light.
- Set a timer to take regular breaks from your desk.
- Use a standing desk when you have the energy.
- Go upstairs to the loo.
- Stand on one leg when you brush your teeth.
- Stand when you use your phone.

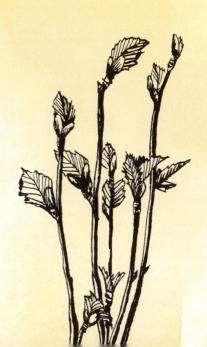

NATURE TIME

Nature is the greatest teacher, especially in the autumnal perimenopause fog, when nothing is clear. Any kind of contact with nature is good – even a photograph of trees can lift your mood – but best of all is to go outside and consciously choose to connect with nature, because this brings us directly into a relationship with the seasons and invites trust and belonging. Embrace the annual seasons – there is always reassurance and beauty to be found, but I can especially recommend you lean into the beauty of annual Autumn as a support to your perimenopause process.

Nature treasures

You can do this little act of nature worship in the park, or a garden, in the countryside, or even with a humble pot plant. Whether you're sitting or walking, put away your phone and settle yourself quietly. Open yourself to nature and follow the curiosity of your senses to connect with the world around you. Drink in the colour, texture and smell of the nature around you, feel the air on your skin, allow yourself to be delighted by the treasures in your environment.

Gratitude

Expressing gratitude is a simple route into a deeper sense of connection and belonging. At its simplest you might say 'thank you' as you pass a tree, but you might want to develop it further by writing a letter, creating an artwork, or performing a gesture or acts of service to the environment around you.

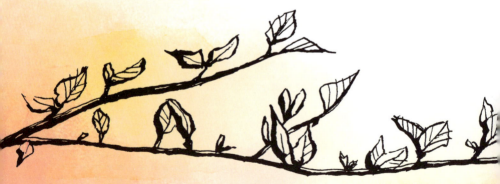

Special friends

Notice which plants and/or locations you are particularly drawn to and give yourself the opportunity to get to know them better, one-to-one. Sit next to them. Listen to them and notice how your system responds. Watch them through the seasons and absorb their wisdom. Engage with your special friend as you would a wise teacher, with respect, compassion and patience, and see what emerges in your relationship.

Gather precious finds to take home and place where they will remind you of the rhythm of the seasons.

Make a cyclical mandala, placing objects to represent each season in each quadrant.

Spring self-care at a glance

When you feel wobbly in Spring, imagine how you might protect and care for yourself as you would a shy child.

SPRING CHALLENGES

Spring is easily missed altogether unless you can slow down a bit before the headlong rush into Summer activity. The hurry to be productive effectively knocks out the gifts of Spring, leaving us afraid of dreaming the impossible dream for fear it gets crushed. Look out for increased anxiety and the surfacing of old trauma which can worsen when you're depleted. A depleted body is not playful or open to adventures.

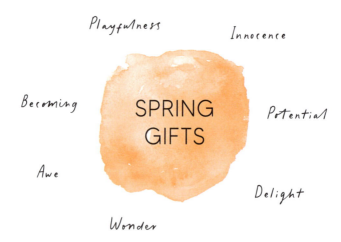

Playfulness

Innocence

Becoming

SPRING GIFTS

Potential

Awe

Delight

Wonder

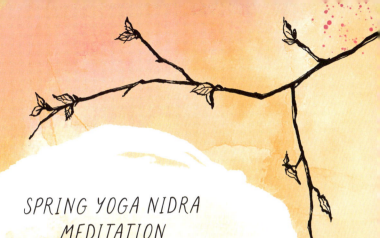

SPRING YOGA NIDRA MEDITATION

Once you've got really comfy and settled in to your resting place, a nidra for Spring invites you to connect with a feeling of gratitude before taking a journey of curiosity and wonder through your body. Immerse yourself in an exploration of groundedness and expansion, followed by a sensory experience of the precious new growth to integrate the Spring qualities of playfulness, innocence, potential, wonder and delight. You can transition from your nidra nest back towards the everyday with the help of the textures and sounds of daily life.

Check in with your inner seasons regularly through the day. You could do it when you brush your teeth, before you eat or when you pick up your phone.

To listen to the yoga nidra, simply scan this QR code on your smartphone and choose from the audio files on offer.

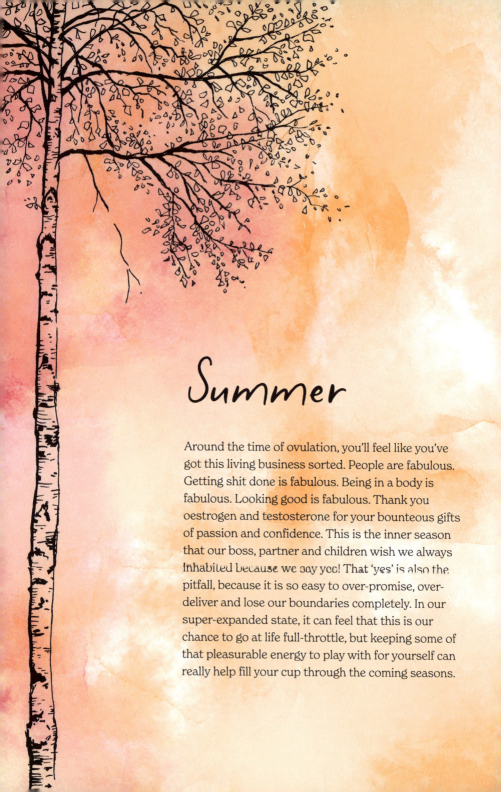

Summer

Around the time of ovulation, you'll feel like you've got this living business sorted. People are fabulous. Getting shit done is fabulous. Being in a body is fabulous. Looking good is fabulous. Thank you oestrogen and testosterone for your bounteous gifts of passion and confidence. This is the inner season that our boss, partner and children wish we always inhabited because we say yes! That 'yes' is also the pitfall, because it is so easy to over-promise, over-deliver and lose our boundaries completely. In our super-expanded state, it can feel that this is our chance to go at life full-throttle, but keeping some of that pleasurable energy to play with for yourself can really help fill your cup through the coming seasons.

SUMMER SELF-CARE

Pleasure

A daily dose of 'vitamin P' supports all mental and physical health.

Grounding

Reduce overwhelm with your preferred grounding practice.

Food

Regular protein and 'upping' micro-nutrients is a must.

Saying yes...

... to yourself! Affirm, validate, reward and celebrate your perfectly imperfect brilliance.

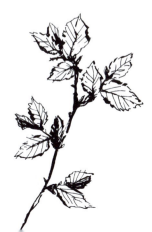

REDUCE EXPECTATIONS

Is your daily to-do list too 'ambitious'? Even back-to-back could it really be done in one day? We constantly expect more than is reasonable and end up judging ourselves as failing.

We habitually take on roles too. For example, the social queen that always organises a mates' night out; the one who's always there when a friend is down. Then there's maintaining a clean-ish home, with bills paid, while holding down a job, looking fresh, with absolutely no freakin' chin hairs. It's impossible to stay sane with this weight of expectations, then you add in perimenopause and there's no way all of this is ever going to happen. While you can't change the expectations of those around you (too exhausting), you can change your own. Luckily in your Autumns you have easy access to your editing capacity. Your NO is available. You can see where there's injustice. You can delegate, reframe, simplify or drop parts of life that are too much. For example, I hate doing the laundry. For years I furiously matched socks, but now all laundry sits in a tangly heap at the top of the stairs and they figure it out themselves.

Now is the natural time to notice where we waste energy so that we can bring it back for ourselves.

Ask yourself

What area of life do you feel most stressed by?

How could you reduce your expectations?

Top tips

I shall be bold here and state that if you're in perimenopause and you have kids, you are going to be feeling guilty that you're not doing enough, especially if they are primary age or younger. So how can we care for ourselves in this situation? The compromise is to balance the Summer parenting demands with a dose of Autumn sensibility. For example:

- Delegate care of or reduce expectations of mess and dirt.

- Reduce the time spent in noisy places full of manic children.

- Connect with your kids with quieter more restful activities.

- Introduce them to the seasons so they can start to learn about rest and self-care.

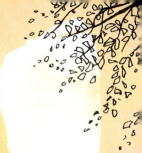

FOOD FOR THOUGHT

You already know that processed food is not your friend and that a Mediterranean diet is widely recommended. Be kind to yourself by gently reducing processed food, increasing the good stuff and forgiving yourself for everything else. Shortest diet book ever.

What's not so widely understood is how stress and emotional eating patterns affect the way we metabolise and absorb nourishment. The main player in perimenopause weight gain is not a lack of self-control, it is stress.

Perimenopause is asking you to emotionally declutter: shed the toxic patterns around food so you can have a vibrant, healthy Second Spring.

Ask yourself

When you were growing up, what words and moods were present around food, eating and body shape? What was the atmosphere at mealtimes?

How do these experiences play out in your life today?

What words or phrases would have been more nourishing for you to hear as a child?

Can you use this information to set an intention?

How was vulnerability met when you were a child?

If these patterns show up in your life now, how can you soothe yourself more appropriately?

Eating for perimenopause wellbeing

- Slow everything down.
- Use your senses to take in the colours, smells and tastes. Chew 10 times or more.
- Reduce stress at mealtimes by turning off your screen.

PACING

Pacing is the art of slowing TF down. You know those people who seem serene and apparently glide through life? That's pacing. We nearly all long for a slower pace of life, but it's tough. The speed at which we are expected to move through life is already too fast and getting faster. But at perimenopause, and in any autumnal or wintery state, we long to slow down – indeed we have to slow down to allow for the recovery and regenerative processes that are on offer here.

As the youngest of three, I always felt I was not quick enough and that there was someone tooting their horn behind me to get a shift on. But through perimenopause I learned to trust that my internal pacing was essential for my wellbeing, and that my constantly rushing to catch up was making me ill. These days, there are times when I am a tortoise just pootling along, and times when I'm the hare, talking at 100mph with my shirt-tails flying. Both are fine because I trust that it's ok to fly, and then ok to rest in turn. Seasonal awareness has taught me to expect to need pacing, most especially after an episode of inner Summer mania.

Pacing might look like...

- Walking more slowly.

- Leaving more space between meetings and events.

- Becoming aware of and stopping the numb-scrolling between activities.

- Eating more slowly.

- Leaving more space before you speak.

- Driving more slowly.

- Letting go of stuff happening when you think it should: self-imposed deadlines? Postpone. Reschedule.

- Saying no to things more often.

- Being late sometimes; being early sometimes too.

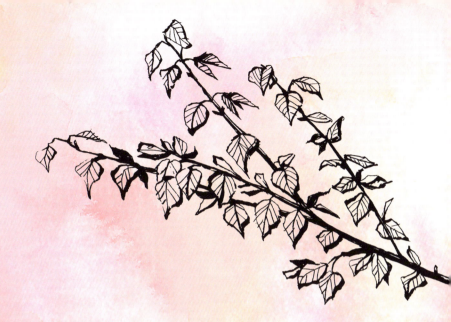

Ask yourself

Reflecting on the previous 24 hours, where did you feel rushed?

If you were to live these 24 hours again at a pace to suit you, what could you change?

What small changes could you make in your life that would support your preferred pace?

Summer self-care at a glance

If you are struggling in Summer, look for how you might be able to celebrate yourself. Even the smallest 'yay' can make a difference.

SUMMER CHALLENGES

It's easy to overwhelm yourself with commitments,
leading to busted boundaries and mania. For sensitive
types and neurodiverse folk, Summer can be a freakin'
nightmare. Too bright, too loud, altogether too much
stimulation, which can tip you into overwhelm and
associated anxiety, depression or disassociation.

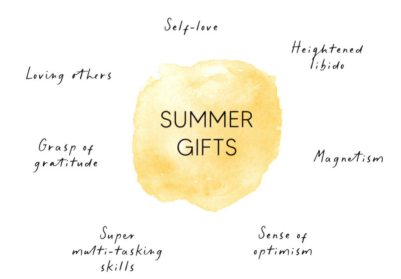

Self-love

Heightened
libido

Loving others

SUMMER
GIFTS

Grasp of
gratitude

Magnetism

Super
multi-tasking
skills

Sense of
optimism

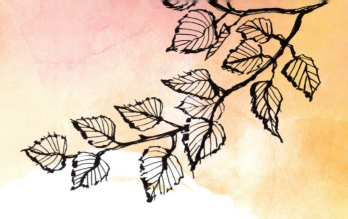

SUMMER YOGA NIDRA MEDITATION

Who doesn't love resting on a Summer's day?
Using the weight of the body to create a safe,
grounded environment, try a guided adventure
that invites pleasure to the body, from the crown
of your head to the tips of your toes. It's great to
use a nidra like this when you're ovulating, wanting
to celebrate yourself, or if you're overwhelmed
by too much 'people time'. You may explore the
contrasting sensations of vibrancy and peace,
and enjoy a sensual experience of Summer
to integrate this season's qualities of flow,
activity, magnetism, energy and connection.

Summer is a great time to have all those difficult
conversations arising from the truths you saw
in Autumn. You are just so much nicer!

To listen to the yoga nidra, simply scan this QR code on
your smartphone and choose from the audio files on offer.

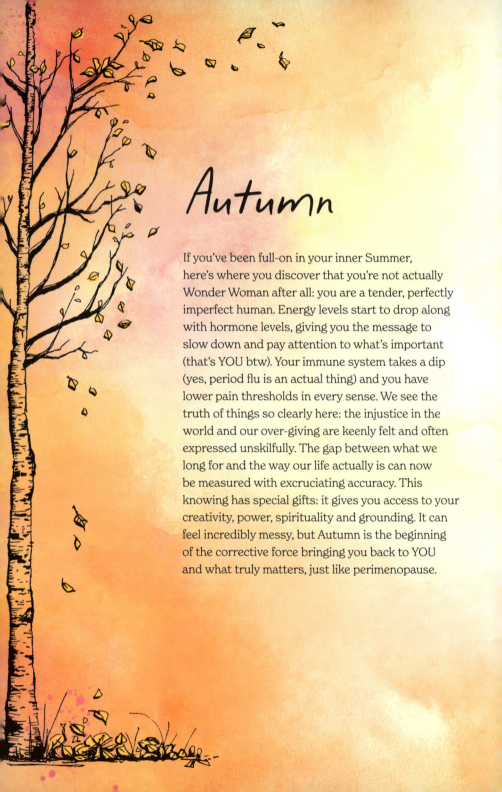

Autumn

If you've been full-on in your inner Summer, here's where you discover that you're not actually Wonder Woman after all: you are a tender, perfectly imperfect human. Energy levels start to drop along with hormone levels, giving you the message to slow down and pay attention to what's important (that's YOU btw). Your immune system takes a dip (yes, period flu is an actual thing) and you have lower pain thresholds in every sense. We see the truth of things so clearly here: the injustice in the world and our over-giving are keenly felt and often expressed unskilfully. The gap between what we long for and the way our life actually is can now be measured with excruciating accuracy. This knowing has special gifts: it gives you access to your creativity, power, spirituality and grounding. It can feel incredibly messy, but Autumn is the beginning of the corrective force bringing you back to YOU and what truly matters, just like perimenopause.

AUTUMN SELF-CARE

Space

Socially distance for your emotional wellbeing. Even a moment to yourself or a walk round the block can save your sanity.

Kindness

Ask, 'What kindness would I love to receive now?' to bring a little more softness and ease into play.

Reducing expectations

No one has as high expectations of you as you do yourself. Lower the bar and let yourself off the hook.

Letting go

Editing is one of Autumn's super-powers and you may find that any kind of clearing, tidying or editing activity will help you reclaim agency.

Enforcing boundaries

You will now be noticing where your boundaries need reassessing.

Trust

Your inner compass is easy to read in Autumn. Listen to that inner knowing to develop trust in your intuition.

SETTING BOUNDARIES

If you've been socialised as female when young, it's likely no one taught you how to say no. How many of you were told to kiss Uncle Bob and not make a fuss, even though you knew it didn't feel safe to do so? Probably you've had to figure out how to set appropriate boundaries along the way. Add in perimenopause exhaustion and a lifetime of saying yes, and we can tend towards either being steamrollered or exploding in a messy refusal. Learning to say no now will take a bit of effort, and prove a super-useful skill. With women doing more housework than men in 93% of heterosexual households, it's clear we've been socialised out of setting boundaries at home too. We have to set boundaries in order to regain our sanity.

Ask Yourself

Recall a time when you said no to something when you were small and describe what happened. What did this teach you about setting boundaries?

What is currently making you feel drained, exploited or violated? These are likely the areas that need a change of boundary.

Bringing to mind something that's a definite no, notice the effect this has on your body – get specific on where you feel tight or small.

Bringing to mind something that's a definite yes, notice the effect this has on your body – get specific on where you feel open or expanded. In everyday life, start to clock these signals; learn to trust and act on them.

What values are important to you? Identify your top three.

What self-care might help you hold a healthy boundary? For example, managing your blood sugar (being hangry tends to put everything on the wonk); getting more rest; talking it through with a friend first; doing strengthening exercises; feeling your legs and feet?

Top tips

- Use 'I' statements that don't criticise or blame the person asking.

- Allow yourself time to ponder an offer before you say yes or no.

- Less is more: you don't have to explain or apologise.

- Every no is a yes to yourself!

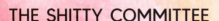

THE SHITTY COMMITTEE

You might feel that you're totally losing the plot with the self-criticism and shaming that goes on in your head, but you're not. We all have it! May I introduce you to what nutritionist Hannah B Burton calls the 'itty bitty shitty committee', aka the inner critic. Ironically the inner critic is trying to protect you from harm by shitting you up and keeping you small to stay safe. Plus a gazillion years of women being regarded as weak and inconsistent doesn't help. But these voices are simply part of being human.

You can banish an inner critic for a while, but the more you try to shut them up the louder they get, so an approach is required which demonstrates that this awful voice is not speaking the truth, and that you are separate from it.

Ask Yourself

Set a timer and freewrite a conversation with your inner critic (you can always tear the page up and bin it later). If you are lucky enough to have a safe, compassionate friend or a professional to consult, you could share your critic's voice with them.

Interrogate your critic. Ask: Is this really true? What do you need from me? What if I don't or can't do what you demand? How could we work better together? Self-compassion and a kind voice are your best defences against a critic attack. You might enquire: What would my best friend advise in this situation? Would I say this to someone I cared about?

Give your critic a name, visualise them as human, creature or alien. Imagine, doodle or draw them.

Find regular grounding practices that work for you: breath awareness, relaxation (drop those shoulders) or yoga nidra are great ways to start. Find some loving, kindly phrases that really hit the spot for you, to use in emergencies – perhaps: 'You're doing so well, my lovely' or 'Just showing up today is more than enough, sweetheart'.

Top tips for wrangling the inner critic

- Don't go near them hangry.
- Make a power playlist of tracks that make you feel invincible.
- Share your achievements, big or small, in your journal or with friends.
- Compliment someone else: your brain responds positively whether you give or receive compliments.

DIGITAL TOXICITY

We live a very different life to our mothers: 100% busier and with 100% more information coming at us all the time. We cannot respond to all the emails and messages that come in. That FOMO feeling grabbing at your ankles is for real. There will always be more podcasts, cat videos, reels and Ted Talks than you will ever be able to watch.

Our screens, though valuable for connection, are also making us stupid: reliance on Google Maps, the super-fast pace, the endless comparisons, are changing our brains and rewiring our nervous systems. It's not our fault – they are designed to be addictive. Perimenopause, with its autumnal call for quiet, insists that we examine our relationship with our phones. The endless parade of lithe, wrinkle-free, white bodies leads to endless unfavourable comparison and frankly the growing, inspirational 'peri-posse' of influencers can be depressing too.

People. It's time to address your relationship with your phone.

Ask yourself

For the rest of today, whenever you notice the impulse to pick up your phone, notice your seasonal and emotional tone.

How can you address this unmet emotional need in your life? For example, if you pick up your phone because you're anxious about your kid, how can you ground yourself and alter your parenting boundaries?

Use this information to set an intention for the upcoming month.

Phone use for perimenopause wellbeing

- Check out the many apps that regulate or restrict phone use

- Set some time boundaries: decide on your daily 'phone hours' and change your settings to 'do not disturb' outside of those. Or better still, turn it off – so liberating!

- Go for a walk without your phone.

- Once a month, even for a day, try deleting your most addictive app.

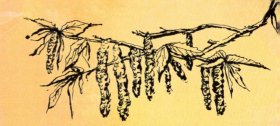

KINDNESS ON THE GO

Kindness on the go is the Deliveroo or UberEats of mindfulness. It's for those moments when you're freaking out, raging, or in total fog-lost-slack-jawed nowhere, and you're desperate for a lifeline. Quite simply, it's about making a small step away from your situation to enquire into what kindness might be supportive. It might be:

- Moving further away from the Zoom screen.

- Giving yourself a moment to stare out of the window.

- Saying 'I'll get back to you on that' in response to a request.

- Putting on your happiest outfit 'just because'.

- Absorbing some texture in your environment through your gaze or touch.

These small kindnesses soothe our nervous systems just enough to give us a little more room to manoeuvre so we can make a better choice. When the only reasonable answer seems to be 'leave and burn it all to the ground' (which it often is), can you step away just a little and give yourself a moment? Navigating perimenopause asks us to balance our inner needs with outer demands and this requires access to a well of compassion within us. But when the well is dry, and we can't find kindness for ourselves, it's time to bring in the special forces. This is when we ponder 'What would my best friend advise here?' or call in anyone whose values you admire. Brene Brown? Tara Brach? Pema Chodron? Let's try it now.

Ask yourself

Let your eyes soften. Exhale through your mouth or sigh, and bring your attention to your heart or belly. Now ask yourself, 'What kindness would I love to receive right now?' and see what comes to you. Then again, a deepening enquiry: 'What do I really need?'

Autumn self-care at a glance

Slow everything down and listen – your inner world is speaking to you.

AUTUMN CHALLENGES

Autumn has a terrible reputation: she is 'problematic'. She is problematic because she announces the change from being a 'good girl' to being yourself. Masking isn't worth it any more – thank goodness for the great corrective that is Autumn. The critics, both inner and outer, can be very loud, along with strong emotions and a sense of feeling lost, so you'll need to call in all your self-care.

Truth telling

Increased discernment

Clearer boundaries

Coming closer to your true values

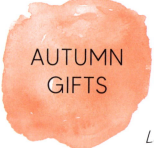

AUTUMN GIFTS

Prioritising yourself over others

More awareness of your needs

Letting go of what no longer serves you

Powerful convictions and strength of feeling

Capacity to organise, edit, and sort stuff out

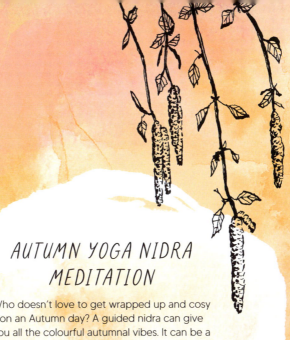

AUTUMN YOGA NIDRA MEDITATION

Who doesn't love to get wrapped up and cosy on an Autumn day? A guided nidra can give you all the colourful autumnal vibes. It can be a support at any time in your perimenopause, but particularly when you're plagued by your inner critic. An Autumn walk around the body invites us to let go at each point, allowing a beautiful release when times are tense. The spirit of Autumn invites you to connect with increased discernment, knowing your truth, understanding what you need, feeling your power before coming back rested and refreshed to greet your day.

All the challenges and self-care of the premenstrual Autumn directly translate into perimenopause.

To listen to the yoga nidra, simply scan this QR code on your smartphone and choose from the audio files on offer.

The inner seasons of perimenopause

Now let's bring perimenopause into the mix. Oh wow! Thanks to fluctuating levels of oestrogen and lower progesterone, you are now in an unknown country, for which there is no definitive test. In fact FSH levels, which prompt the ovaries into action, fluctuate so much it's not possible to definitively show perimenopause, only early menopause or postmenopause. So let's leave the measuring of our hormones for now – far better to *feel* our way into the seasons and address those.

What most people experience when hormones start to fluctuate in perimenopause is more Autumn and Winter vibes. This might mean, if you're experiencing longer cycles, the premenstrual time goes on and on and on; or for some, there's more of an autumnal cloud that occupies the whole of their cycle, 'dulling out' the Spring and Summer. As Autumn advances you might start to wonder 'where's sexy gone?' because in some cycles you won't ovulate at all. It does not mean that sex is over, it just means that we change from a physiological response to eroticism, to what pleasures us deeply. What does this mean in real life? More sensitivity, stronger feelings, lower energy and a lot less tolerance for other people taking bloody liberties. Think premenstrual for the longest time.

You can see why, for those lucky enough to have followed their cycle with menstrual season awareness, they'll have built up an excellent Autumn toolkit before perimenopause arrives. But even if, like me, you haven't got into the awesome power of the inner seasons before you arrive in your perimenopause, here is your training ground! You are being asked to slow

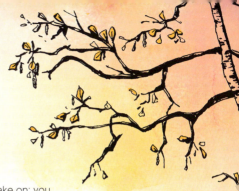

down and be more discerning about what you take on: you will learn to delegate, you will be brought round to be kinder to yourself in all sorts of ways, and over time these things will become non-negotiable.

As the rhythm of predictable inner seasons shifts, it's time to level up and become an inner season ninja so you can spot the different seasons as they show up in your daily life. They will still be there, just in a different form. For example, a sunny early morning filled with possibilities = Spring; flirty eye contact = Summer. You can call on the quality and the self-care of each season to guide you through your daily life. This intuitive approach is so simple and it cuts through a lot that can trip us up: over-thinking, self-judgement, shame and disassociation. Incidentally, you'll often find guides to the inner seasons giving you specific days when they'll be there, which is particularly unhelpful in perimenopause. These guides only show what you could expect in the average person, not the actual terrain of messy, real life. Only you can tell where you are. This seasonal approach is offering you the key to your authority. It is regular checking in and reflection on what season you relate to, and how you can care for yourself, that will open the lock.

Autumn sensitivity gives an opportunity for old wounds and patterns to be healed, so expect some strong feelings here. Try to welcome them and allow them to move through you so you can release and heal.

How to Use This Journal

I invite you to start where you're at. Right now, crack open the first page of the journal part of this book and write today's date on the appropriate day of the week. Then just note down how you're feeling, any emotions that are dominating, and your energy levels. That's it. Life is complicated and overwhelming, so keep it as simple as you can. For extra points, add in what season you feel you may be in, your cycle day and the moon phase, but only when you have the energy; the act of noting how you are is more than enough.

Your menstrual cycle will be on the move in perimenopause, growing shorter or longer and maybe skipping months at a time. It's a good idea to drop the expectation of a 28-day-ish rhythm, and instead just notice the season you feel most closely aligned to each day. This means that the weekly journalling pages may not match your menstrual rhythm, and that's ok. It's all about grounding yourself in your experience as you transition to a new way of being. As my teacher Alexandra Pope says, after the rhythm of the menstrual cycle has gone 'the training wheels are off'!

It is very confusing understanding what is causing your symptoms – is it perimenopause or is it life stress? Trauma or blood sugar? As complex beings touched by systemic injustice, environmental pollutions, conditioning, genetics and relationships, let alone what we had for breakfast, it's no wonder there's an addiction to overthinking. You may never know the true cause, but you can care for yourself as you are. By responding to the season you feel most connected to in the moment, you can instantly soothe your nervous system and reduce stress. This seasonal kindness will help you stay in touch with your feelings, communicate and strategise, and provide yourself with the best care for most of the mental and physical conditions you're grappling with. Top side-benefit? You are role-modelling excellent self-care for your kids, friends, colleagues and family and giving them permission to do the same. It's not all about you (even though it actually is)!

Now you've read through the descriptions of the seasons and the self-care prompts, and rested with yoga nidra, as you continue noting down how you feel each day, you'll easily start to identify how the seasons feel to you. Each day has a space for seasonal self-care: this is where you can record what helps you from day to day. Over time this will build your tool kit of care for each season. Don't forget you can check out a yoga nidra meditation whenever you feel like it, so you can integrate your understanding of the seasons while lying down and having a rest; no effort required.

The journal pages have been laid out to give maximum flexibility for you to record what is important for you. Please go crazy with coloured pens, doodles, stickers and words in any way that pleases you. If it's not fun and pleasurable, it's never going to be a consistent habit, so do it your way.

On the weekly journal pages there's space to fill in the date, moon phase and menstrual day so that you can keep an eye out for cyclical lunar and menstrual patterns. Next there's space for you to record the seasons you noticed through your day and underneath that, your seasonal self-care. This is your place to lay it all out and get naked with yourself; all kinds of ranting and enquiry are welcomed as well as tracking what the hell's going on. The focus will change over time, so alongside your investigation into your seasons, you might be tracking:

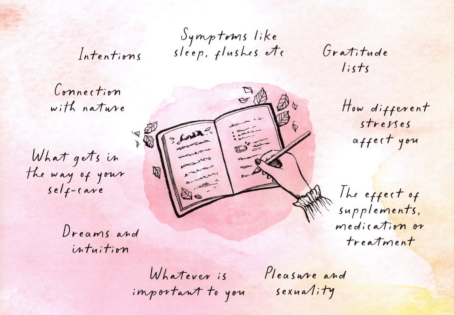

Intentions

Symptoms like sleep, flushes etc

Gratitude lists

Connection with nature

How different stresses affect you

What gets in the way of your self-care

The effect of supplements, medication or treatment

Dreams and intuition

Whatever is important to you

Pleasure and sexuality

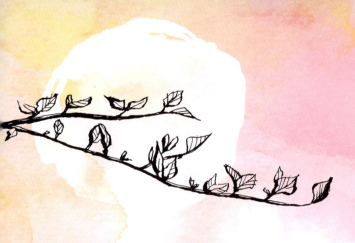

Intentions of all kinds benefit from repetition to affirm and hold your focus, so there's space for setting those at the start of the journal, and for reflecting and revising them at the end of each four-week cycle. You'll also find a moon chart for each cycle. See the Setting Intentions & Reflecting and the Moon Charts sections that follow for a bit of guidance.

Release yourself from any expectations of filling in everything every week. We have all had five-year diaries in the back of the cupboard entirely blank except for two pages. Do what you can, in a way that is kind and helps you understand your inner seasons. Your journal entry can be as simple as a cross or a tick.

Just as no two perimenopause experiences are the same, so your needs are absolutely unique, so go with what feels truthful and useful for you. Another important aspect is that the themes you track will change over time: for example, you might be interested in tracking the connection between sugar and the emotions you're struggling with for a month or two, then that will fade and you might get into meditation, or moving more. When your tracking shifts, that's really ok. Be kind to yourself and let things go when you need to, follow what interests you and if in doubt, track your vulnerabilities and how you can better care for them. Please don't use this journal as another place to beat yourself up and find yourself wanting. Goodness knows there are enough places that will do this for you. Let this be a place of curiosity, reflection and yes, that sticky, gooey self-love.

No need to overthink it – just using a plus or minus sign can be enough to make connections.

Setting intentions & reflecting

Intention setting is a helpful way to keep you steady as you navigate the choppy waters of perimenopause. We're not talking about pushing towards goals here, but a quality of being – less 'lose 10lbs by Christmas', and more 'treat my body with kindness'. An intention should be stated in the positive, and you can set them either as your period draws to an end, or with the new moon. You might like to journal about it based on what's arisen in the previous weeks, or let it come to you when you go for a walk in nature. If you want to get boujee with it, you can make a ritual of it by lighting a candle as you write or saying your intentions aloud.

At the end of each week there's space for reflection. Reflecting on what you are proud of builds self-worth. Some days this might be getting out of pyjamas, saying no, or adding in an extra portion of vegetables to your dinner. The benefits are doubled because as well as celebrating yourself, you can also look back through them when you're having a wobbly day and remember all the wonderful things about yourself.

Looking at what new things are emerging is another great way to keep yourself on track, so at the bottom of each weekly page there's a space to record anything new. It might be celebrating new habits, observing patterns of overwhelm, or noticing where you sabotage yourself. No judgements though! Just noticing the changes that are occurring is more than enough because the other weekly reflection is 'What can I let go of?' This might be a belief, draining tasks or anything that's not serving you in your life. These reflections naturally bring you to what intentions you'd like to create for the coming month.

Hindsight is a wonderful thing and your journalling is going to give you this in spades. You'll find that a little distance can bring clarity that is inaccessible when you're in the thick of things. Whenever you need perspective, flip back through a month or two to see what has changed. Full of self-hatred? Check out what you have been proud of. In a complete freeze and don't know what to do? Peruse your growing library of seasonal self-care to remember what might feel good.

Intentions meditation

I've created a meditation which you can download to support your monthly intention setting – just scan the QR code in Audio Guides for Meditation in The Seasons section of this book.

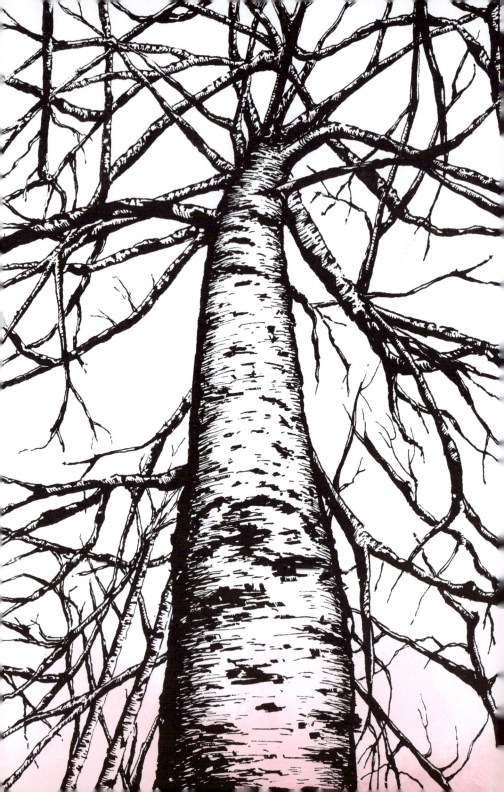

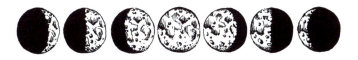

Moon charts

Though our second favourite lump of rock is a million miles away, she exerts an enormous pull on the earth. At the full moon, corals on the Great Barrier Reef release a mass spawning event, and all over the world people can't sleep. We are all more or less affected by the moon cycle, so it's helpful to know what the moon's up to as we chart our own experiences. An app will tell you what the current moon phase is, but wherever possible, go outside and look at the actual moon. Getting to know the different phases and trajectories truly roots us into the rhythm of life. Many find that everything gets more intense at the full moon, and has a quieter more introverted vibe close to the new moon.

On the first page of the journal section of this book you'll find a circular cycle chart for each month. This can provide an alternative way to begin noticing your unique patterns and themes because you only have a small space to write a few words in.

HOW TO USE THE MOON CHARTS

The moon charts are a quick way to track symptoms and how the moon may be playing into your energy levels and sensitivities. You can use them when time is short and you're not able to use the journal pages, or in parallel with your daily reflections to deepen your awareness. Here's what to do:

1. Find out when the last new moon was, and put the date at the top of the chart.

2. Mark the dates clockwise in the appropriate spaces.

3. In today's segment, in the 'flow' space, note any period, discharge or cervical fluid.

4. Then in today's 'feelings' space note your energy level, emotions and anything else that feels important to track.

5. Don't forget to check back and observe any patterns at the end of the month.

The example here of a partially filled-in moon chart may give you some ideas about what you would like to record on your own charts. Feel free to own the process with colour, stickers or whatever floats your boat, and track what is important to you. As part of your monthly reflections, have a look back at the previous months' charts and check for patterns and shifts. When you can observe regular responses to the moon, use these to plan your activities to enhance the different qualities available to you. Note: the moon phases around the edge are only a guide and may not fit what's happening in the sky, as moon cycles vary from month to month. Before electric light and Netflix we would all have felt the effect of the moon, and regulated ourselves accordingly, so as part of your practice try to check in with the actual moon as often as you can.

Date of new moon...   Monday 11th Jan 2024

Dates go here

New moon date

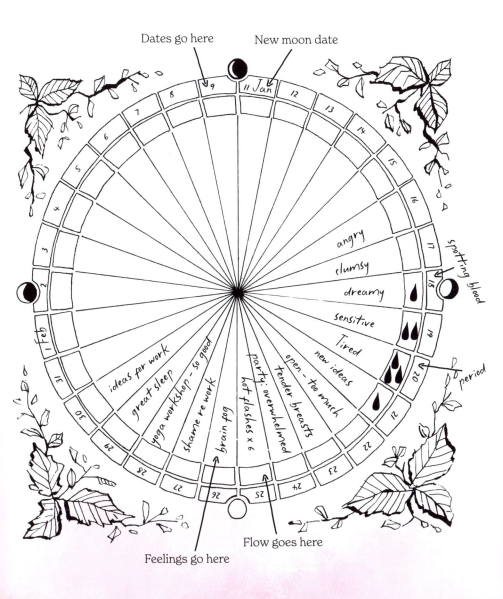

11 Jan

angry
clumsy
dreamy
sensitive
tired
new ideas

open – too much
tender breasts
party: overwhelmed
hot flashes x 6
brain fog
shame re work
yoga workshop – so good
great sleep
ideas for work

spotting blood

period

Flow goes here

Feelings go here

Your Journal

TIME TO GET STARTED

Let's get real here: it's only in the realms of fantasy that we have ample time for journalling every day. In real life, we may just be able to scribble a word or two, and that's absolutely fine. If you only have a tiny moment to yourself right now, turn to the first journal page and just note how you feel. This small act is more than enough; the power of witnessing yourself, even for a moment, is huge. If you can gift yourself a little longer, try this:

Take a moment to exhale and settle yourself. Maybe place one hand on your belly and the other on your heart. Get curious about sensations in your body, notice your thoughts as they come and go, and as the swirl of impressions lands, ask yourself, 'What season do I most identify with right now?' and jot it down. Then ask, 'What would I love to receive right now?' and write it down – there's your seasonal care right there. If it's a giant need like a month by the sea, and it feels impossible to receive in your lunchbreak, see if you can at least give yourself a 30 second blast of fresh air.

Have fun building your library of self-care. Each kindness you can receive is another step towards a Second Spring.

You are the expert on you!

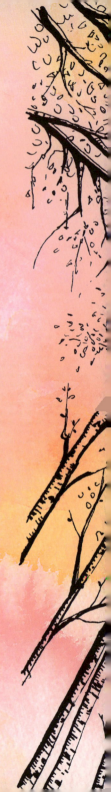

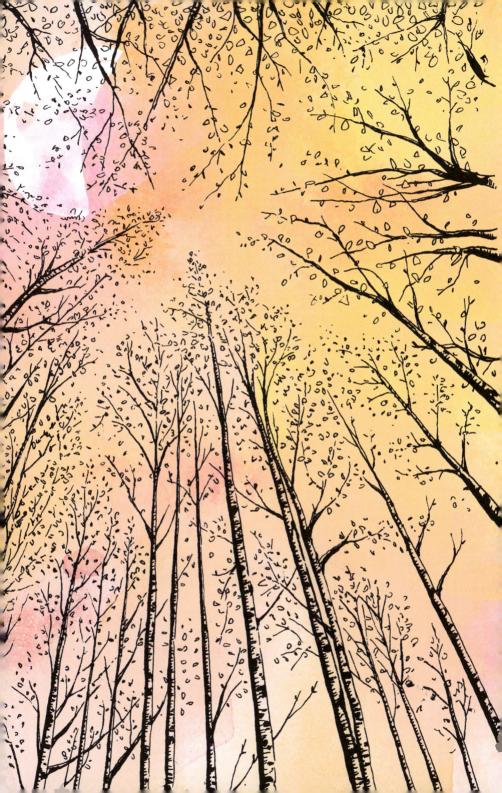

Cycle One

SETTING INTENTIONS

Beginnings equate to springtime and can hold a multitude of different feelings which often pull us in different directions. Whatever is showing up for you right now, you're in a great place to set an intention for yourself. Just acknowledge the rich, complex experience of being yourself as you are today, call in a blanket of kindness, and take a look at Setting Intentions and Reflecting in the How to Use This Journal section of the book, which will help you hone your intentions for the coming weeks.

Jot down some positive intentions here to help you navigate the next four weeks or so...

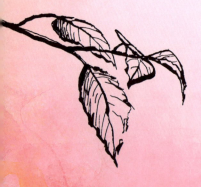

MOON CHART

Date of new moon...

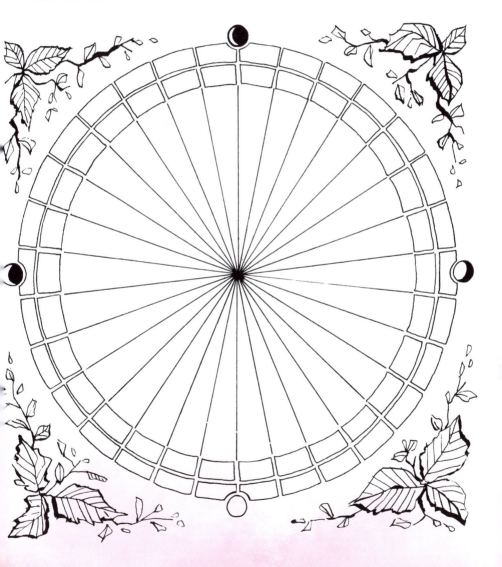

Monday

Date .... Moon phase ◯ Cycle day ....

How am I feeling? ....

What season(s) am I experiencing? ....

Seasonal self-care ....

....

....

Tuesday

Date .... Moon phase ◯ Cycle day ....

How am I feeling? ....

What season(s) am I experiencing? ....

Seasonal self-care ....

....

....

Wednesday

Date .... Moon phase ◯ Cycle day ....

How am I feeling? ....

What season(s) am I experiencing? ....

Seasonal self-care ....

....

....

Thursday

Date .... Moon phase ◯ Cycle day ....

How am I feeling? ....

What season(s) am I experiencing? ....

Seasonal self-care ....

....

....

If in doubt, get out of your own way.

Friday
Date _____ Moon phase ○ Cycle day _____

How am I feeling? _____

What season(s) am I experiencing? _____

Seasonal self-care _____

_____

_____

Saturday
Date _____ Moon phase ○ Cycle day _____

How am I feeling? _____

What season(s) am I experiencing? _____

Seasonal self-care _____

_____

_____

Sunday
Date _____ Moon phase ○ Cycle day _____

How am I feeling? _____

What season(s) am I experiencing? _____

Seasonal self-care _____

_____

_____

Weekly reflections

What's new?

What can I let go of?

Monday   Date _____   Moon phase ◯ Cycle day _____

How am I feeling? _____

What season(s) am I experiencing? _____

Seasonal self-care _____

_____

_____

Tuesday   Date _____   Moon phase ◯ Cycle day _____

How am I feeling? _____

What season(s) am I experiencing? _____

Seasonal self-care _____

_____

_____

Wednesday Date _____   Moon phase ◯ Cycle day _____

How am I feeling? _____

What season(s) am I experiencing? _____

Seasonal self-care _____

_____

_____

Thursday   Date _____   Moon phase ◯ Cycle day _____

How am I feeling? _____

What season(s) am I experiencing? _____

Seasonal self-care _____

_____

_____

Rest is your first aid, time alone is your medicine.

Friday
Date .... Moon phase ◯ Cycle day ....
How am I feeling? ....
What season(s) am I experiencing? ....
Seasonal self-care ....

....
....

Saturday
Date .... Moon phase ◯ Cycle day ....
How am I feeling? ....
What season(s) am I experiencing? ....
Seasonal self-care ....

....
....

Sunday
Date .... Moon phase ◯ Cycle day ....
How am I feeling? ....
What season(s) am I experiencing? ....
Seasonal self-care ....

....
....

Weekly reflections

What's new?

What can I let go of?

Monday   Date ....   Moon phase ◯   Cycle day ....

How am I feeling? ....

What season(s) am I experiencing? ....

Seasonal self-care ....

....

....

Tuesday   Date ....   Moon phase ◯   Cycle day ....

How am I feeling? ....

What season(s) am I experiencing? ....

Seasonal self-care ....

....

....

Wednesday   Date ....   Moon phase ◯   Cycle day ....

How am I feeling? ....

What season(s) am I experiencing? ....

Seasonal self-care ....

....

....

Thursday   Date ....   Moon phase ◯   Cycle day ....

How am I feeling? ....

What season(s) am I experiencing? ....

Seasonal self-care ....

....

....

Take your time: be tender and gentle with yourself.

Friday

Date _____ Moon phase ◯ Cycle day _____

How am I feeling? _____

What season(s) am I experiencing? _____

Seasonal self-care _____

_____

Saturday

Date _____ Moon phase ◯ Cycle day _____

How am I feeling? _____

What season(s) am I experiencing? _____

Seasonal self-care _____

_____

Sunday

Date _____ Moon phase ◯ Cycle day _____

How am I feeling? _____

What season(s) am I experiencing? _____

Seasonal self-care _____

_____

Weekly reflections

What's new?

What can I let go of?

Monday   Date _____   Moon phase ◯   Cycle day

How am I feeling? _____

What season(s) am I experiencing? _____

Seasonal self-care _____

_____

_____

Tuesday   Date _____   Moon phase ◯   Cycle day

How am I feeling? _____

What season(s) am I experiencing? _____

Seasonal self-care _____

_____

_____

Wednesday   Date _____   Moon phase ◯   Cycle day

How am I feeling? _____

What season(s) am I experiencing? _____

Seasonal self-care _____

_____

_____

Thursday   Date _____   Moon phase ◯   Cycle day

How am I feeling? _____

What season(s) am I experiencing? _____

Seasonal self-care _____

_____

_____

What can you feel genuinely grateful for right now?

Friday   Date ....   Moon phase ◯ Cycle day ....

How am I feeling? ....

What season(s) am I experiencing? ....

Seasonal self-care ....

....

....

Saturday   Date ....   Moon phase ◯ Cycle day ....

How am I feeling? ....

What season(s) am I experiencing? ....

Seasonal self-care ....

....

....

Sunday   Date ....   Moon phase ◯ Cycle day ....

How am I feeling? ....

What season(s) am I experiencing? ....

Seasonal self-care ....

....

....

Weekly reflections

What's new?

What can I let go of?

Cycle Two

MONTHLY REFLECTIONS

Four weeks have passed, and you're poised on the brink of a new cycle. Though it might feel like a messy blur to you now, there is so much gold to be found in reflecting on your experiences. Wrap yourself in a blanket of self-love, have a flip through your journal pages from the previous weeks, check in with the Setting Intentions and Reflecting section in How to Use This Journal, and ponder the enquiries below.

What am I really proud of achieving?

What patterns do I notice from my moon chart?

What new things are emerging for me?

What can I let go of?

What intentions can I make for next month?

MOON CHART

Date of new moon...

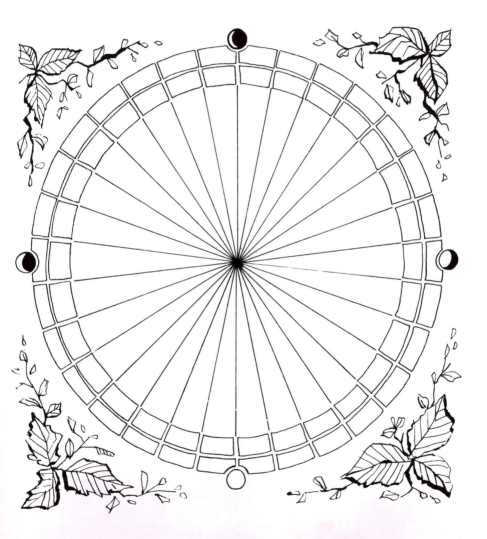

Monday   Date   Moon phase ◯   Cycle day

How am I feeling?

What season(s) am I experiencing?

Seasonal self-care

Tuesday   Date   Moon phase ◯   Cycle day

How am I feeling?

What season(s) am I experiencing?

Seasonal self-care

Wednesday   Date   Moon phase ◯   Cycle day

How am I feeling?

What season(s) am I experiencing?

Seasonal self-care

Thursday   Date   Moon phase ◯   Cycle day

How am I feeling?

What season(s) am I experiencing?

Seasonal self-care

Joy can be found in the most surprising places.

Friday

Date _____   Moon phase ◯   Cycle day _____

How am I feeling? _____

What season(s) am I experiencing? _____

Seasonal self-care _____

_____

Saturday

Date _____   Moon phase ◯   Cycle day _____

How am I feeling? _____

What season(s) am I experiencing? _____

Seasonal self-care _____

_____

Sunday

Date _____   Moon phase ◯   Cycle day _____

How am I feeling? _____

What season(s) am I experiencing? _____

Seasonal self-care _____

_____

Weekly reflections

What's new?

What can I let go of?

Monday　　　Date _____　　Moon phase ◯　Cycle day _____

How am I feeling? _____

What season(s) am I experiencing? _____

Seasonal self-care _____

_____

_____

Tuesday　　　Date _____　　Moon phase ◯　Cycle day _____

How am I feeling? _____

What season(s) am I experiencing? _____

Seasonal self-care _____

_____

_____

Wednesday　Date _____　　Moon phase ◯　Cycle day _____

How am I feeling? _____

What season(s) am I experiencing? _____

Seasonal self-care _____

_____

_____

Thursday　　Date _____　　Moon phase ◯　Cycle day _____

How am I feeling? _____

What season(s) am I experiencing? _____

Seasonal self-care _____

_____

_____

You get to decide what is important.

Friday
Date .... Moon phase ◯ Cycle day ....

How am I feeling? ....

What season(s) am I experiencing? ....

Seasonal self-care ....

Saturday
Date .... Moon phase ◯ Cycle day ....

How am I feeling? ....

What season(s) am I experiencing? ....

Seasonal self-care ....

Sunday
Date .... Moon phase ◯ Cycle day ....

How am I feeling? ....

What season(s) am I experiencing? ....

Seasonal self-care ....

Weekly reflections

What's new?

What can I let go of?

Monday   Date ....   Moon phase ◯ Cycle day ....

How am I feeling? ....

What season(s) am I experiencing? ....

Seasonal self-care ....

....

....

Tuesday   Date ....   Moon phase ◯ Cycle day ....

How am I feeling? ....

What season(s) am I experiencing? ....

Seasonal self-care ....

....

....

Wednesday   Date ....   Moon phase ◯ Cycle day ....

How am I feeling? ....

What season(s) am I experiencing? ....

Seasonal self-care ....

....

....

Thursday   Date ....   Moon phase ◯ Cycle day ....

How am I feeling? ....

What season(s) am I experiencing? ....

Seasonal self-care ....

....

....

If you can't have the nourishment you long for, give yourself a snack-sized version.

Friday
Date .... Moon phase ◯ Cycle day ....

How am I feeling? ....

What season(s) am I experiencing? ....

Seasonal self-care ....

....

....

Saturday
Date .... Moon phase ◯ Cycle day ....

How am I feeling? ....

What season(s) am I experiencing? ....

Seasonal self-care ....

....

....

Sunday
Date .... Moon phase ◯ Cycle day ....

How am I feeling? ....

What season(s) am I experiencing? ....

Seasonal self-care ....

....

....

Weekly reflections

What's new?

What can I let go of?

Monday　　　Date ....　　Moon phase ◯ Cycle day ....

How am I feeling? ....

What season(s) am I experiencing? ....

Seasonal self-care ....

....

....

Tuesday　　　Date ....　　Moon phase ◯ Cycle day ....

How am I feeling? ....

What season(s) am I experiencing? ....

Seasonal self-care ....

....

....

Wednesday　　Date ....　　Moon phase ◯ Cycle day ....

How am I feeling? ....

What season(s) am I experiencing? ....

Seasonal self-care ....

....

....

Thursday　　　Date ....　　Moon phase ◯ Cycle day ....

How am I feeling? ....

What season(s) am I experiencing? ....

Seasonal self-care ....

....

....

Perimenopause is like puberty in reverse — release you inner teen.

Friday   Date .... Moon phase ◯ Cycle day ....

How am I feeling? ....

What season(s) am I experiencing? ....

Seasonal self-care ....

....

Saturday   Date .... Moon phase ◯ Cycle day ....

How am I feeling? ....

What season(s) am I experiencing? ....

Seasonal self-care ....

....

Sunday   Date .... Moon phase ◯ Cycle day ....

How am I feeling? ....

What season(s) am I experiencing? ....

Seasonal self-care ....

....

Weekly reflections

What's new?

What can I let go of?

Cycle Three

MONTHLY REFLECTIONS

Another four weeks have passed, and you're poised on the brink of a new cycle. Though it might feel like a messy blur to you now, there is so much gold to be found in reflecting on your experiences. Wrap yourself in a blanket of self-love, have a flip through your journal pages from the previous weeks, check in with the Setting Intentions and Reflecting section in How to Use This Journal, and ponder the enquiries below.

What am I really proud of achieving?

Looking back at the last two months' moon charts, what patterns are occurring?

What new things are emerging for me?

What can I let go of?

What intentions can I make for next month?

MOON CHART

Date of new moon...

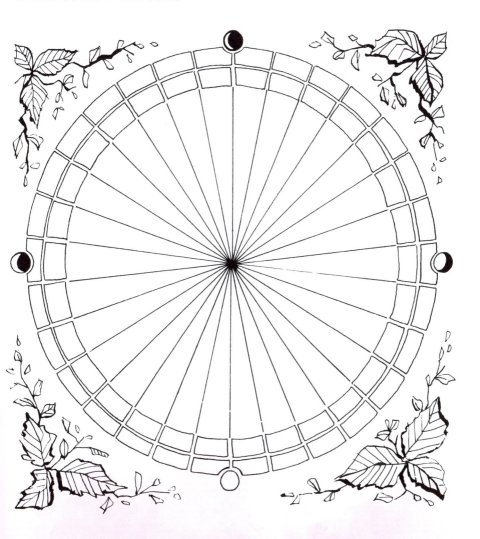

Monday   Date ....   Moon phase ◯ Cycle day ....

How am I feeling? ....

What season(s) am I experiencing? ....

Seasonal self-care ....

....

....

Tuesday   Date ....   Moon phase ◯ Cycle day ....

How am I feeling? ....

What season(s) am I experiencing? ....

Seasonal self-care ....

....

....

Wednesday   Date ....   Moon phase ◯ Cycle day ....

How am I feeling? ....

What season(s) am I experiencing? ....

Seasonal self-care ....

....

....

Thursday   Date ....   Moon phase ◯ Cycle day ....

How am I feeling? ....

What season(s) am I experiencing? ....

Seasonal self-care ....

....

....

Dare to trust there is meaning in everyday life.

Friday   Date _____   Moon phase ◯ Cycle day _____

How am I feeling? _____

What season(s) am I experiencing? _____

Seasonal self-care _____

_____

Saturday   Date _____   Moon phase ◯ Cycle day _____

How am I feeling? _____

What season(s) am I experiencing? _____

Seasonal self-care _____

_____

Sunday   Date _____   Moon phase ◯ Cycle day _____

How am I feeling? _____

What season(s) am I experiencing? _____

Seasonal self-care _____

_____

Weekly reflections

What's new?

What can I let go of?

Monday   Date   Moon phase ◯ Cycle day

How am I feeling?

What season(s) am I experiencing?

Seasonal self-care

Tuesday   Date   Moon phase ◯ Cycle day

How am I feeling?

What season(s) am I experiencing?

Seasonal self-care

Wednesday   Date   Moon phase ◯ Cycle day

How am I feeling?

What season(s) am I experiencing?

Seasonal self-care

Thursday   Date   Moon phase ◯ Cycle day

How am I feeling?

What season(s) am I experiencing?

Seasonal self-care

You're the authority on you: no one else can know what you really need.

Friday
Date .... Moon phase ◯ Cycle day ....

How am I feeling? ....

What season(s) am I experiencing? ....

Seasonal self-care ....

....

Saturday
Date .... Moon phase ◯ Cycle day ....

How am I feeling? ....

What season(s) am I experiencing? ....

Seasonal self-care ....

....

Sunday
Date .... Moon phase ◯ Cycle day ....

How am I feeling? ....

What season(s) am I experiencing? ....

Seasonal self-care ....

....

Weekly reflections

What's new?

What can I let go of?

Monday   Date _____   Moon phase ○   Cycle day _____

How am I feeling? _____

What season(s) am I experiencing? _____

Seasonal self-care _____

_____

_____

Tuesday   Date _____   Moon phase ○   Cycle day _____

How am I feeling? _____

What season(s) am I experiencing? _____

Seasonal self-care _____

_____

_____

Wednesday   Date _____   Moon phase ○   Cycle day _____

How am I feeling? _____

What season(s) am I experiencing? _____

Seasonal self-care _____

_____

_____

Thursday   Date _____   Moon phase ○   Cycle day _____

How am I feeling? _____

What season(s) am I experiencing? _____

Seasonal self-care _____

_____

_____

You do not have to justify or explain your needs. Ever.

Friday
Date _____ Moon phase ◯ Cycle day _____

How am I feeling? _____

What season(s) am I experiencing? _____

Seasonal self-care _____

_____

_____

Saturday
Date _____ Moon phase ◯ Cycle day _____

How am I feeling? _____

What season(s) am I experiencing? _____

Seasonal self-care _____

_____

_____

Sunday
Date _____ Moon phase ◯ Cycle day _____

How am I feeling? _____

What season(s) am I experiencing? _____

Seasonal self-care _____

_____

_____

Weekly reflections

What's new?

What can I let go of?

Monday

Date .... Moon phase ◯ Cycle day ....

How am I feeling? ....

What season(s) am I experiencing? ....

Seasonal self-care ....

....

....

Tuesday

Date .... Moon phase ◯ Cycle day ....

How am I feeling? ....

What season(s) am I experiencing? ....

Seasonal self-care ....

....

....

Wednesday

Date .... Moon phase ◯ Cycle day ....

How am I feeling? ....

What season(s) am I experiencing? ....

Seasonal self-care ....

....

....

Thursday

Date .... Moon phase ◯ Cycle day ....

How am I feeling? ....

What season(s) am I experiencing? ....

Seasonal self-care ....

....

....

Even the tiniest act of self-care makes a difference.

Friday

Date _____ Moon phase ◯ Cycle day _____

How am I feeling? _____

What season(s) am I experiencing? _____

Seasonal self-care _____

_____

Saturday

Date _____ Moon phase ◯ Cycle day _____

How am I feeling? _____

What season(s) am I experiencing? _____

Seasonal self-care _____

_____

Sunday

Date _____ Moon phase ◯ Cycle day _____

How am I feeling? _____

What season(s) am I experiencing? _____

Seasonal self-care _____

_____

Weekly reflections

What's new?

What can I let go of?

Cycle Four

MONTHLY REFLECTIONS

Another four weeks have passed, and you're poised on the brink of a new cycle. Though it might feel like a messy blur to you now, there is so much gold to be found in reflecting on your experiences. Wrap yourself in a blanket of self-love, have a flip through your journal pages from the previous weeks, check in with the Setting Intentions and Reflecting section in How to Use This Journal, and ponder the enquiries below.

What am I really proud of achieving?

Looking back at the last few months' moon charts, what patterns are occurring?

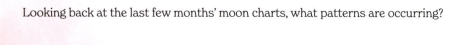

What new things are emerging for me?

What can I let go of?

What intentions can I make for next month?

MOON CHART

Date of new moon...

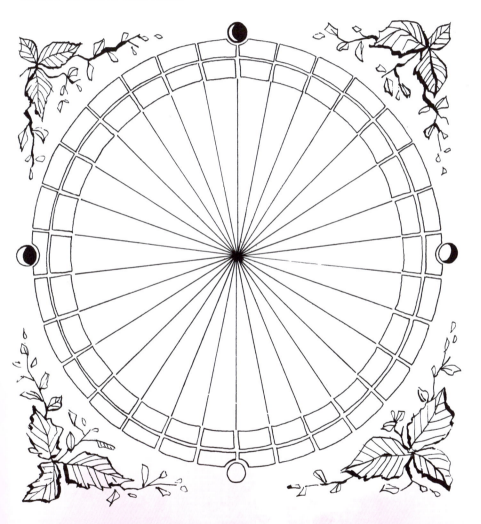

Monday Date .... Moon phase ◯ Cycle day ....

How am I feeling? ....

What season(s) am I experiencing? ....

Seasonal self-care ....

....

....

Tuesday Date .... Moon phase ◯ Cycle day ....

How am I feeling? ....

What season(s) am I experiencing? ....

Seasonal self-care ....

....

....

Wednesday Date .... Moon phase ◯ Cycle day ....

How am I feeling? ....

What season(s) am I experiencing? ....

Seasonal self-care ....

....

....

Thursday Date .... Moon phase ◯ Cycle day ....

How am I feeling? ....

What season(s) am I experiencing? ....

Seasonal self-care ....

....

....

What can you celebrate about yourself today?

Friday

Date _____   Moon phase ◯   Cycle day _____

How am I feeling? _____

What season(s) am I experiencing? _____

Seasonal self-care _____

_____

_____

Saturday

Date _____   Moon phase ◯   Cycle day _____

How am I feeling? _____

What season(s) am I experiencing? _____

Seasonal self-care _____

_____

_____

Sunday

Date _____   Moon phase ◯   Cycle day _____

How am I feeling? _____

What season(s) am I experiencing? _____

Seasonal self-care _____

_____

_____

Weekly reflections

What's new?

What can I let go of?

Monday   Date ....   Moon phase ◯ Cycle day ....

How am I feeling? ....

What season(s) am I experiencing? ....

Seasonal self-care ....

....

....

Tuesday   Date ....   Moon phase ◯ Cycle day ....

How am I feeling? ....

What season(s) am I experiencing? ....

Seasonal self-care ....

....

....

Wednesday   Date ....   Moon phase ◯ Cycle day ....

How am I feeling? ....

What season(s) am I experiencing? ....

Seasonal self-care ....

....

....

Thursday   Date ....   Moon phase ◯ Cycle day ....

How am I feeling? ....

What season(s) am I experiencing? ....

Seasonal self-care ....

....

....

Everything unfolds at its own pace and in its own unique way, including you.

Friday

Date .... Moon phase ◯ Cycle day ....

How am I feeling? ....

What season(s) am I experiencing? ....

Seasonal self-care ....

....

Saturday

Date .... Moon phase ◯ Cycle day ....

How am I feeling? ....

What season(s) am I experiencing? ....

Seasonal self-care ....

....

Sunday

Date .... Moon phase ◯ Cycle day ....

How am I feeling? ....

What season(s) am I experiencing? ....

Seasonal self-care ....

....

Weekly reflections

What's new?

What can I let go of?

Monday   Date ....   Moon phase ◯ Cycle day ....

How am I feeling? ....

What season(s) am I experiencing? ....

Seasonal self-care ....

....

....

Tuesday   Date ....   Moon phase ◯ Cycle day ....

How am I feeling? ....

What season(s) am I experiencing? ....

Seasonal self-care ....

....

....

Wednesday Date ....   Moon phase ◯ Cycle day ....

How am I feeling? ....

What season(s) am I experiencing? ....

Seasonal self-care ....

....

....

Thursday   Date ....   Moon phase ◯ Cycle day ....

How am I feeling? ....

What season(s) am I experiencing? ....

Seasonal self-care ....

....

....

Your body already knows how to do perimenopause.

Friday
Date _____ Moon phase ◯ Cycle day _____

How am I feeling? _____

What season(s) am I experiencing? _____

Seasonal self-care _____

_____

Saturday
Date _____ Moon phase ◯ Cycle day _____

How am I feeling? _____

What season(s) am I experiencing? _____

Seasonal self-care _____

_____

Sunday
Date _____ Moon phase ◯ Cycle day _____

How am I feeling? _____

What season(s) am I experiencing? _____

Seasonal self-care _____

_____

Weekly reflections

What's new?

What can I let go of?

Monday   Date _____   Moon phase ◯ Cycle day _____

How am I feeling? _____

What season(s) am I experiencing? _____

Seasonal self-care _____

_____

_____

Tuesday   Date _____   Moon phase ◯ Cycle day _____

How am I feeling? _____

What season(s) am I experiencing? _____

Seasonal self-care _____

_____

_____

Wednesday   Date _____   Moon phase ◯ Cycle day _____

How am I feeling? _____

What season(s) am I experiencing? _____

Seasonal self-care _____

_____

_____

Thursday   Date _____   Moon phase ◯ Cycle day _____

How am I feeling? _____

What season(s) am I experiencing? _____

Seasonal self-care _____

_____

_____

Let go of trying to get back to who you used to be: relax into who you are now.

Friday   Date ....   Moon phase ◯ Cycle day ....

How am I feeling? ....

What season(s) am I experiencing? ....

Seasonal self-care ....

....

....

Saturday   Date ....   Moon phase ◯ Cycle day ....

How am I feeling? ....

What season(s) am I experiencing? ....

Seasonal self-care ....

....

....

Sunday   Date ....   Moon phase ◯ Cycle day ....

How am I feeling? ....

What season(s) am I experiencing? ....

Seasonal self-care ....

....

....

Weekly reflections

What's new?

What can I let go of?

Cycle Five

MONTHLY REFLECTIONS

Another four weeks have passed, and you're poised on the brink of a new cycle. Though it might feel like a messy blur to you now, there is so much gold to be found in reflecting on your experiences. Wrap yourself in a blanket of self-love, have a flip through your journal pages from the previous weeks, check in with the Setting Intentions and Reflecting section in How to Use This Journal, and ponder the enquiries below.

What am I really proud of achieving?

Looking back at the last few months' moon charts, what patterns are occurring?

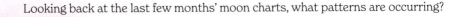

What new things are emerging for me?

What can I let go of?

What intentions can I make for next month?

MOON CHART

Date of new moon...

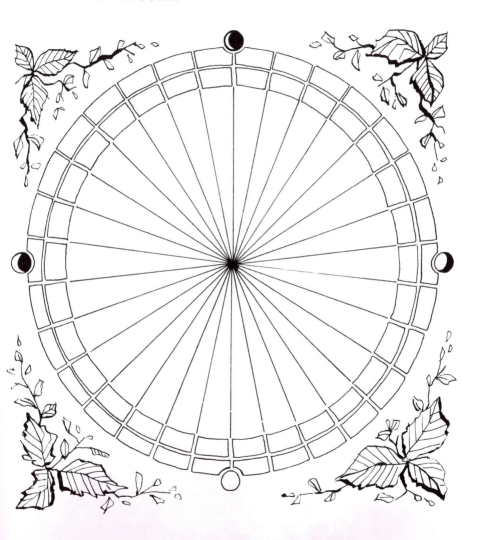

Monday   Date ....   Moon phase ◯ Cycle day ....

How am I feeling? ....

What season(s) am I experiencing? ....

Seasonal self-care ....

....

....

Tuesday   Date ....   Moon phase ◯ Cycle day ....

How am I feeling? ....

What season(s) am I experiencing? ....

Seasonal self-care ....

....

....

Wednesday   Date ....   Moon phase ◯ Cycle day ....

How am I feeling? ....

What season(s) am I experiencing? ....

Seasonal self-care ....

....

....

Thursday   Date ....   Moon phase ◯ Cycle day ....

How am I feeling? ....

What season(s) am I experiencing? ....

Seasonal self-care ....

....

....

Honour your boundaries as a gift to celebrate yourself.

Friday

Date .... Moon phase ◯ Cycle day ....

How am I feeling? ....

What season(s) am I experiencing? ....

Seasonal self-care ....

....

....

Saturday

Date .... Moon phase ◯ Cycle day ....

How am I feeling? ....

What season(s) am I experiencing? ....

Seasonal self-care ....

....

....

Sunday

Date .... Moon phase ◯ Cycle day ....

How am I feeling? ....

What season(s) am I experiencing? ....

Seasonal self-care ....

....

....

Weekly reflections

What's new?

What can I let go of?

Monday   Date   Moon phase ◯   Cycle day

How am I feeling?

What season(s) am I experiencing?

Seasonal self-care

Tuesday   Date   Moon phase ◯   Cycle day

How am I feeling?

What season(s) am I experiencing?

Seasonal self-care

Wednesday   Date   Moon phase ◯   Cycle day

How am I feeling?

What season(s) am I experiencing?

Seasonal self-care

Thursday   Date   Moon phase ◯   Cycle day

How am I feeling?

What season(s) am I experiencing?

Seasonal self-care

Let softness and spaciousness be your first step in the face of challenges.

Friday
Date .... Moon phase ◯ Cycle day ....

How am I feeling? ....

What season(s) am I experiencing? ....

Seasonal self-care ....

....

....

Saturday
Date .... Moon phase ◯ Cycle day ....

How am I feeling? ....

What season(s) am I experiencing? ....

Seasonal self-care ....

....

....

Sunday
Date .... Moon phase ◯ Cycle day ....

How am I feeling? ....

What season(s) am I experiencing? ....

Seasonal self-care ....

....

....

Weekly reflections

What's new?

What can I let go of?

Monday   Date _____   Moon phase ◯ Cycle day _____

How am I feeling? _____

What season(s) am I experiencing? _____

Seasonal self-care _____

_____

_____

Tuesday   Date _____   Moon phase ◯ Cycle day _____

How am I feeling? _____

What season(s) am I experiencing? _____

Seasonal self-care _____

_____

_____

Wednesday   Date _____   Moon phase ◯ Cycle day _____

How am I feeling? _____

What season(s) am I experiencing? _____

Seasonal self-care _____

_____

_____

Thursday   Date _____   Moon phase ◯ Cycle day _____

How am I feeling? _____

What season(s) am I experiencing? _____

Seasonal self-care _____

_____

_____

There is no medal for muscling through without support.

Friday Date .... Moon phase ◯ Cycle day ....

How am I feeling? ....

What season(s) am I experiencing? ....

Seasonal self-care ....

....

....

Saturday Date .... Moon phase ◯ Cycle day ....

How am I feeling? ....

What season(s) am I experiencing? ....

Seasonal self-care ....

....

....

Sunday Date .... Moon phase ◯ Cycle day ....

How am I feeling? ....

What season(s) am I experiencing? ....

Seasonal self-care ....

....

....

Weekly reflections

What's new?

What can I let go of?

Monday   Date ....   Moon phase ◯ Cycle day ....

How am I feeling? ....

What season(s) am I experiencing? ....

Seasonal self-care ....

....

....

Tuesday   Date ....   Moon phase ◯ Cycle day ....

How am I feeling? ....

What season(s) am I experiencing? ....

Seasonal self-care ....

....

....

Wednesday   Date ....   Moon phase ◯ Cycle day ....

How am I feeling? ....

What season(s) am I experiencing? ....

Seasonal self-care ....

....

....

Thursday   Date ....   Moon phase ◯ Cycle day ....

How am I feeling? ....

What season(s) am I experiencing? ....

Seasonal self-care ....

....

....

How can you love yourself better today?

Friday
Date .... Moon phase ◯ Cycle day ....

How am I feeling? ....

What season(s) am I experiencing? ....

Seasonal self-care ....

....

....

Saturday
Date .... Moon phase ◯ Cycle day ....

How am I feeling? ....

What season(s) am I experiencing? ....

Seasonal self-care ....

....

....

Sunday
Date .... Moon phase ◯ Cycle day ....

How am I feeling? ....

What season(s) am I experiencing? ....

Seasonal self-care ....

....

....

Weekly reflections

What's new?

What can I let go of?

Cycle Six

MONTHLY REFLECTIONS

Another four weeks have passed, and you're poised on the brink of a new cycle. Though it might feel like a messy blur to you now, there is so much gold to be found in reflecting on your experiences. Wrap yourself in a blanket of self-love, have a flip through your journal pages from the previous weeks, check in with the Setting Intentions and Reflecting section in How to Use This Journal, and ponder the enquiries below.

What am I really proud of achieving?

Looking back at the last few months' moon charts, what patterns are occurring?

What new things are emerging for me?

What can I let go of?

What intentions can I make for next month?

MOON CHART

Date of new moon...

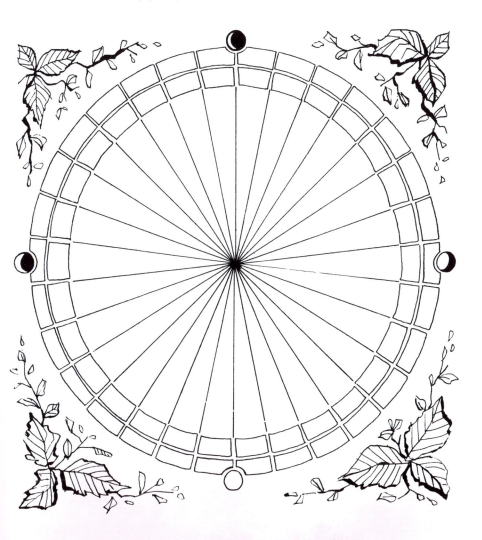

Monday   Date ....   Moon phase ◯ Cycle day ....

How am I feeling? ....

What season(s) am I experiencing? ....

Seasonal self-care ....

....

....

Tuesday   Date ....   Moon phase ◯ Cycle day ....

How am I feeling? ....

What season(s) am I experiencing? ....

Seasonal self-care ....

....

....

Wednesday   Date ....   Moon phase ◯ Cycle day ....

How am I feeling? ....

What season(s) am I experiencing? ....

Seasonal self-care ....

....

....

Thursday   Date ....   Moon phase ◯ Cycle day ....

How am I feeling? ....

What season(s) am I experiencing? ....

Seasonal self-care ....

....

....

What might be the kindest option for you right now?

Friday
Date .... Moon phase ◯ Cycle day ....

How am I feeling? ....

What season(s) am I experiencing? ....

Seasonal self-care ....

....

Saturday
Date .... Moon phase ◯ Cycle day ....

How am I feeling? ....

What season(s) am I experiencing? ....

Seasonal self-care ....

....

Sunday
Date .... Moon phase ◯ Cycle day ....

How am I feeling? ....

What season(s) am I experiencing? ....

Seasonal self-care ....

....

Weekly reflections

What's new?

What can I let go of?

Monday   Date _____   Moon phase ◯   Cycle day _____

How am I feeling? _____

What season(s) am I experiencing? _____

Seasonal self-care _____

_____

_____

Tuesday   Date _____   Moon phase ◯   Cycle day _____

How am I feeling? _____

What season(s) am I experiencing? _____

Seasonal self-care _____

_____

_____

Wednesday   Date _____   Moon phase ◯   Cycle day _____

How am I feeling? _____

What season(s) am I experiencing? _____

Seasonal self-care _____

_____

_____

Thursday   Date _____   Moon phase ◯   Cycle day _____

How am I feeling? _____

What season(s) am I experiencing? _____

Seasonal self-care _____

_____

_____

Write yourself a permission slip to do absolutely nothing.

Friday

Date _____ Moon phase ◯ Cycle day _____

How am I feeling? _____

What season(s) am I experiencing? _____

Seasonal self-care _____

_____

_____

Saturday

Date _____ Moon phase ◯ Cycle day _____

How am I feeling? _____

What season(s) am I experiencing? _____

Seasonal self-care _____

_____

_____

Sunday

Date _____ Moon phase ◯ Cycle day _____

How am I feeling? _____

What season(s) am I experiencing? _____

Seasonal self-care _____

_____

_____

Weekly reflections

What's new?

What can I let go of?

Monday   Date   Moon phase ◯   Cycle day

How am I feeling?

What season(s) am I experiencing?

Seasonal self-care

Tuesday   Date   Moon phase ◯   Cycle day

How am I feeling?

What season(s) am I experiencing?

Seasonal self-care

Wednesday   Date   Moon phase ◯   Cycle day

How am I feeling?

What season(s) am I experiencing?

Seasonal self-care

Thursday   Date   Moon phase ◯   Cycle day

How am I feeling?

What season(s) am I experiencing?

Seasonal self-care

Your feelings are valid.

Friday   Date   Moon phase ◯ Cycle day

How am I feeling?

What season(s) am I experiencing?

Seasonal self-care

Saturday   Date   Moon phase ◯ Cycle day

How am I feeling?

What season(s) am I experiencing?

Seasonal self-care

Sunday   Date   Moon phase ◯ Cycle day

How am I feeling?

What season(s) am I experiencing?

Seasonal self-care

Weekly reflections

What's new?

What can I let go of?

Monday   Date   Moon phase ◯ Cycle day

How am I feeling?

What season(s) am I experiencing?

Seasonal self-care

Tuesday   Date   Moon phase ◯ Cycle day

How am I feeling?

What season(s) am I experiencing?

Seasonal self-care

Wednesday   Date   Moon phase ◯ Cycle day

How am I feeling?

What season(s) am I experiencing?

Seasonal self-care

Thursday   Date   Moon phase ◯ Cycle day

How am I feeling?

What season(s) am I experiencing?

Seasonal self-care

It's not you: the world is not organised to support cyclical beings.

Friday   Date ....   Moon phase ◯ Cycle day ....

How am I feeling? ....

What season(s) am I experiencing? ....

Seasonal self-care ....

....

....

Saturday   Date ....   Moon phase ◯ Cycle day ....

How am I feeling? ....

What season(s) am I experiencing? ....

Seasonal self-care ....

....

....

Sunday   Date ....   Moon phase ◯ Cycle day ....

How am I feeling? ....

What season(s) am I experiencing? ....

Seasonal self-care ....

....

....

Weekly reflections

What's new?

What can I let go of?

Cycle Seven

MONTHLY REFLECTIONS

Another four weeks have passed, and you're poised on the brink of a new cycle. Though it might feel like a messy blur to you now, there is so much gold to be found in reflecting on your experiences. Wrap yourself in a blanket of self-love, have a flip through your journal pages from the previous weeks, check in with the Setting Intentions and Reflecting section in How to Use This Journal, and ponder the enquiries below.

What am I really proud of achieving?

Looking back at the last few months' moon charts, what patterns are occurring?

What new things are emerging for me?

What can I let go of?

What intentions can I make for next month?

MOON CHART

Date of new moon...

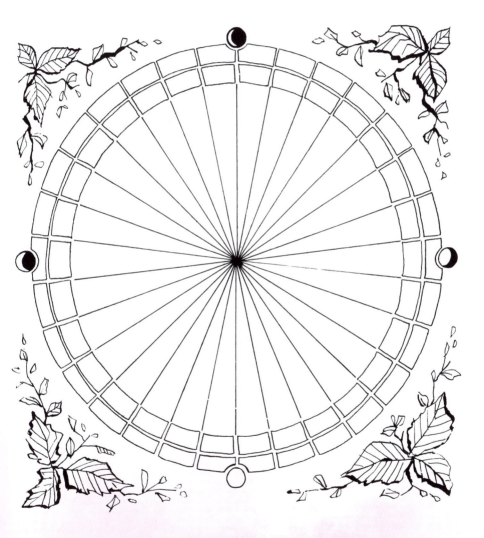

Monday   Date _____   Moon phase ◯ Cycle day _____

How am I feeling? _____

What season(s) am I experiencing? _____

Seasonal self-care _____

_____

_____

Tuesday   Date _____   Moon phase ◯ Cycle day _____

How am I feeling? _____

What season(s) am I experiencing? _____

Seasonal self-care _____

_____

_____

Wednesday   Date _____   Moon phase ◯ Cycle day _____

How am I feeling? _____

What season(s) am I experiencing? _____

Seasonal self-care _____

_____

_____

Thursday   Date _____   Moon phase ◯ Cycle day _____

How am I feeling? _____

What season(s) am I experiencing? _____

Seasonal self-care _____

_____

_____

Cyclical renewal is often dismissed as 'inconsistency' by people who don't get it.

Friday   Date ....   Moon phase ◯   Cycle day ....

How am I feeling? ....

What season(s) am I experiencing? ....

Seasonal self-care ....

....

....

Saturday   Date ....   Moon phase ◯   Cycle day ....

How am I feeling? ....

What season(s) am I experiencing? ....

Seasonal self-care ....

....

....

Sunday   Date ....   Moon phase ◯   Cycle day ....

How am I feeling? ....

What season(s) am I experiencing? ....

Seasonal self-care ....

....

....

Weekly reflections

What's new?

What can I let go of?

Monday   Date   Moon phase ◯ Cycle day

How am I feeling?

What season(s) am I experiencing?

Seasonal self-care

Tuesday   Date   Moon phase ◯ Cycle day

How am I feeling?

What season(s) am I experiencing?

Seasonal self-care

Wednesday Date   Moon phase ◯ Cycle day

How am I feeling?

What season(s) am I experiencing?

Seasonal self-care

Thursday   Date   Moon phase ◯ Cycle day

How am I feeling?

What season(s) am I experiencing?

Seasonal self-care

Kindness is required in all seasons.

Friday
Date _____   Moon phase ◯   Cycle day _____

How am I feeling? _____

What season(s) am I experiencing? _____

Seasonal self-care _____

_____

_____

Saturday
Date _____   Moon phase ◯   Cycle day _____

How am I feeling? _____

What season(s) am I experiencing? _____

Seasonal self-care _____

_____

_____

Sunday
Date _____   Moon phase ◯   Cycle day _____

How am I feeling? _____

What season(s) am I experiencing? _____

Seasonal self-care _____

_____

_____

Weekly reflections

What's new?

What can I let go of?

Monday   Date ....   Moon phase ⃝ Cycle day ....

How am I feeling? ....

What season(s) am I experiencing? ....

Seasonal self-care ....

....

....

Tuesday   Date ....   Moon phase ⃝ Cycle day ....

How am I feeling? ....

What season(s) am I experiencing? ....

Seasonal self-care ....

....

....

Wednesday   Date ....   Moon phase ⃝ Cycle day ....

How am I feeling? ....

What season(s) am I experiencing? ....

Seasonal self-care ....

....

....

Thursday   Date ....   Moon phase ⃝ Cycle day ....

How am I feeling? ....

What season(s) am I experiencing? ....

Seasonal self-care ....

....

....

Autumnal rage can give you an idea of your power and potency.

Friday
Date .... Moon phase ◯ Cycle day ....

How am I feeling? ....

What season(s) am I experiencing? ....

Seasonal self-care ....

....

Saturday
Date .... Moon phase ◯ Cycle day ....

How am I feeling? ....

What season(s) am I experiencing? ....

Seasonal self-care ....

....

Sunday
Date .... Moon phase ◯ Cycle day ....

How am I feeling? ....

What season(s) am I experiencing? ....

Seasonal self-care ....

....

Weekly reflections

What's new?

What can I let go of?

Monday   Date ....   Moon phase ◯ Cycle day ....

How am I feeling? ....

What season(s) am I experiencing? ....

Seasonal self-care ....

....

....

Tuesday   Date ....   Moon phase ◯ Cycle day ....

How am I feeling? ....

What season(s) am I experiencing? ....

Seasonal self-care ....

....

....

Wednesday   Date ....   Moon phase ◯ Cycle day ....

How am I feeling? ....

What season(s) am I experiencing? ....

Seasonal self-care ....

....

....

Thursday   Date ....   Moon phase ◯ Cycle day ....

How am I feeling? ....

What season(s) am I experiencing? ....

Seasonal self-care ....

....

....

What feels like an emergency may actually be
the emergence of a new way of being.

Friday

Date .... Moon phase ◯ Cycle day ....

How am I feeling? ....

What season(s) am I experiencing? ....

Seasonal self-care ....

....

Saturday

Date .... Moon phase ◯ Cycle day ....

How am I feeling? ....

What season(s) am I experiencing? ....

Seasonal self-care ....

....

Sunday

Date .... Moon phase ◯ Cycle day ....

How am I feeling? ....

What season(s) am I experiencing? ....

Seasonal self-care ....

....

Weekly reflections

What's new?

What can I let go of?

Cycle Eight

MONTHLY REFLECTIONS

Another four weeks have passed, and you're poised on the brink of a new cycle. Though it might feel like a messy blur to you now, there is so much gold to be found in reflecting on your experiences. Wrap yourself in a blanket of self-love, have a flip through your journal pages from the previous weeks, check in with the Setting Intentions and Reflecting section in How to Use This Journal, and ponder the enquiries below.

What am I really proud of achieving?

Looking back at the last few months' moon charts, what patterns are occurring?

What new things are emerging for me?

What can I let go of?

What intentions can I make for next month?

MOON CHART

Date of new moon...

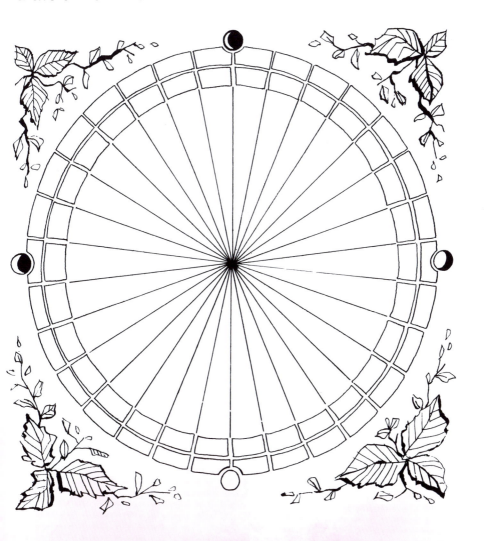

Monday
Date .... Moon phase ◯ Cycle day ....

How am I feeling? ....

What season(s) am I experiencing? ....

Seasonal self-care ....

....

....

Tuesday
Date .... Moon phase ◯ Cycle day ....

How am I feeling? ....

What season(s) am I experiencing? ....

Seasonal self-care ....

....

....

Wednesday
Date .... Moon phase ◯ Cycle day ....

How am I feeling? ....

What season(s) am I experiencing? ....

Seasonal self-care ....

....

....

Thursday
Date .... Moon phase ◯ Cycle day ....

How am I feeling? ....

What season(s) am I experiencing? ....

Seasonal self-care ....

....

....

Autumn brings the change from being 'good' to being yourself.

Friday   Date ....   Moon phase ◯ Cycle day ....

How am I feeling? ....

What season(s) am I experiencing? ....

Seasonal self-care ....

....

....

Saturday   Date ....   Moon phase ◯ Cycle day ....

How am I feeling? ....

What season(s) am I experiencing? ....

Seasonal self-care ....

....

....

Sunday   Date ....   Moon phase ◯ Cycle day ....

How am I feeling? ....

What season(s) am I experiencing? ....

Seasonal self-care ....

....

....

Weekly reflections

What's new?

What can I let go of?

Monday   Date ....   Moon phase ◯   Cycle day ....

How am I feeling? ....

What season(s) am I experiencing? ....

Seasonal self-care ....

....

....

Tuesday   Date ....   Moon phase ◯   Cycle day ....

How am I feeling? ....

What season(s) am I experiencing? ....

Seasonal self-care ....

....

....

Wednesday   Date ....   Moon phase ◯   Cycle day ....

How am I feeling? ....

What season(s) am I experiencing? ....

Seasonal self-care ....

....

....

Thursday   Date ....   Moon phase ◯   Cycle day ....

How am I feeling? ....

What season(s) am I experiencing? ....

Seasonal self-care ....

....

....

Validate yourself: every achievement, from tiny to huge, is worthy of celebration.

Friday   Date ....   Moon phase ◯ Cycle day ....

How am I feeling? ....

What season(s) am I experiencing? ....

Seasonal self-care ....

....

Saturday   Date ....   Moon phase ◯ Cycle day ....

How am I feeling? ....

What season(s) am I experiencing? ....

Seasonal self-care ....

....

Sunday   Date ....   Moon phase ◯ Cycle day ....

How am I feeling? ....

What season(s) am I experiencing? ....

Seasonal self-care ....

....

Weekly reflections

What's new?

What can I let go of?

Monday   Date ....   Moon phase $\bigcirc$ Cycle day ....

How am I feeling? ....

What season(s) am I experiencing? ....

Seasonal self-care ....

....

....

Tuesday   Date ....   Moon phase $\bigcirc$ Cycle day ....

How am I feeling? ....

What season(s) am I experiencing? ....

Seasonal self-care ....

....

....

Wednesday   Date ....   Moon phase $\bigcirc$ Cycle day ....

How am I feeling? ....

What season(s) am I experiencing? ....

Seasonal self-care ....

....

....

Thursday   Date ....   Moon phase $\bigcirc$ Cycle day ....

How am I feeling? ....

What season(s) am I experiencing? ....

Seasonal self-care ....

....

....

What might it mean to say YES to yourself today?

Friday   Date _____   Moon phase ◯ Cycle day _____

How am I feeling? ....

What season(s) am I experiencing? ....

Seasonal self-care ....

....

....

Saturday   Date _____   Moon phase ◯ Cycle day _____

How am I feeling? ....

What season(s) am I experiencing? ....

Seasonal self-care ....

....

....

Sunday   Date _____   Moon phase ◯ Cycle day _____

How am I feeling? ....

What season(s) am I experiencing? ....

Seasonal self-care ....

....

....

Weekly reflections

What's new?

What can I let go of?

Monday   Date _____   Moon phase ◯   Cycle day _____

How am I feeling? _____

What season(s) am I experiencing? _____

Seasonal self-care _____

_____

_____

Tuesday   Date _____   Moon phase ◯   Cycle day _____

How am I feeling? _____

What season(s) am I experiencing? _____

Seasonal self-care _____

_____

_____

Wednesday   Date _____   Moon phase ◯   Cycle day _____

How am I feeling? _____

What season(s) am I experiencing? _____

Seasonal self-care _____

_____

_____

Thursday   Date _____   Moon phase ◯   Cycle day _____

How am I feeling? _____

What season(s) am I experiencing? _____

Seasonal self-care _____

_____

_____

Call in protection and forgiveness to ease the vulnerability of Spring.

Friday   Date _____   Moon phase ◯   Cycle day _____

How am I feeling? _____

What season(s) am I experiencing? _____

Seasonal self-care _____

_____

_____

Saturday   Date _____   Moon phase ◯   Cycle day _____

How am I feeling? _____

What season(s) am I experiencing? _____

Seasonal self-care _____

_____

_____

Sunday   Date _____   Moon phase ◯   Cycle day _____

How am I feeling? _____

What season(s) am I experiencing? _____

Seasonal self-care _____

_____

_____

Weekly reflections

What's new?

What can I let go of?

Cycle Nine

MONTHLY REFLECTIONS

Another four weeks have passed, and you're poised on the brink of a new cycle. Though it might feel like a messy blur to you now, there is so much gold to be found in reflecting on your experiences. Wrap yourself in a blanket of self-love, have a flip through your journal pages from the previous weeks, check in with the Setting Intentions and Reflecting section in How to Use This Journal, and ponder the enquiries below.

What am I really proud of achieving?

Looking back at the last few months' moon charts, what patterns are occurring?

What new things are emerging for me?

What can I let go of?

What intentions can I make for next month?

MOON CHART

Date of new moon...

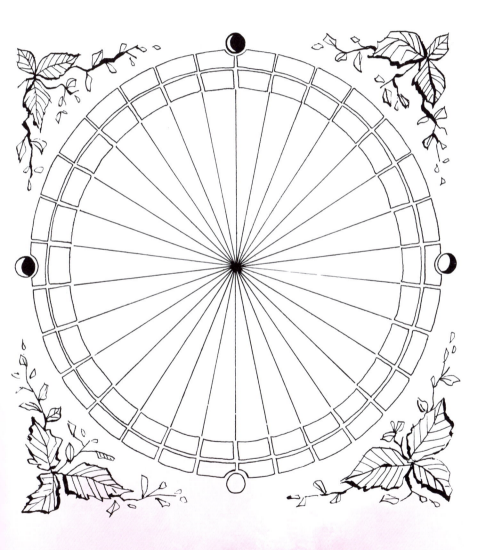

Monday   Date   Moon phase ◯ Cycle day

How am I feeling?

What season(s) am I experiencing?

Seasonal self-care

Tuesday   Date   Moon phase ◯ Cycle day

How am I feeling?

What season(s) am I experiencing?

Seasonal self-care

Wednesday   Date   Moon phase ◯ Cycle day

How am I feeling?

What season(s) am I experiencing?

Seasonal self-care

Thursday   Date   Moon phase ◯ Cycle day

How am I feeling?

What season(s) am I experiencing?

Seasonal self-care

How can you bring more pleasure into your day?

Friday
Date _____   Moon phase ○   Cycle day _____

How am I feeling? _____

What season(s) am I experiencing? _____

Seasonal self-care _____

_____

_____

Saturday
Date _____   Moon phase ○   Cycle day _____

How am I feeling? _____

What season(s) am I experiencing? _____

Seasonal self-care _____

_____

_____

Sunday
Date _____   Moon phase ○   Cycle day _____

How am I feeling? _____

What season(s) am I experiencing? _____

Seasonal self-care _____

_____

_____

Weekly reflections

What's new?

What can I let go of?

Monday   Date ....   Moon phase ◯ Cycle day ....

How am I feeling? ....

What season(s) am I experiencing? ....

Seasonal self-care ....

....

....

Tuesday   Date ....   Moon phase ◯ Cycle day ....

How am I feeling? ....

What season(s) am I experiencing? ....

Seasonal self-care ....

....

....

Wednesday   Date ....   Moon phase ◯ Cycle day ....

How am I feeling? ....

What season(s) am I experiencing? ....

Seasonal self-care ....

....

....

Thursday   Date ....   Moon phase ◯ Cycle day ....

How am I feeling? ....

What season(s) am I experiencing? ....

Seasonal self-care ....

....

....

Running around like an ovulating 20 year old will end up in burnout.

Friday
Date .... Moon phase ◯ Cycle day

How am I feeling? ....

What season(s) am I experiencing? ....

Seasonal self-care ....

....

....

Saturday
Date .... Moon phase ◯ Cycle day

How am I feeling? ....

What season(s) am I experiencing? ....

Seasonal self-care ....

....

....

Sunday
Date .... Moon phase ◯ Cycle day

How am I feeling? ....

What season(s) am I experiencing? ....

Seasonal self-care ....

....

....

Weekly reflections

What's new?

What can I let go of?

Monday   Date   Moon phase ◯ Cycle day
How am I feeling?
What season(s) am I experiencing?
Seasonal self-care

Tuesday   Date   Moon phase ◯ Cycle day
How am I feeling?
What season(s) am I experiencing?
Seasonal self-care

Wednesday   Date   Moon phase ◯ Cycle day
How am I feeling?
What season(s) am I experiencing?
Seasonal self-care

Thursday   Date   Moon phase ◯ Cycle day
How am I feeling?
What season(s) am I experiencing?
Seasonal self-care

Your longing has deep intelligence: it's telling you where to go.

Friday

Date _____   Moon phase ◯   Cycle day _____

How am I feeling? _____

What season(s) am I experiencing? _____

Seasonal self-care _____

_____

Saturday

Date _____   Moon phase ◯   Cycle day _____

How am I feeling? _____

What season(s) am I experiencing? _____

Seasonal self-care _____

_____

Sunday

Date _____   Moon phase ◯   Cycle day _____

How am I feeling? _____

What season(s) am I experiencing? _____

Seasonal self-care _____

_____

Weekly reflections

What's new?

What can I let go of?

Monday   Date   Moon phase ◯ Cycle day

How am I feeling?

What season(s) am I experiencing?

Seasonal self-care

Tuesday   Date   Moon phase ◯ Cycle day

How am I feeling?

What season(s) am I experiencing?

Seasonal self-care

Wednesday   Date   Moon phase ◯ Cycle day

How am I feeling?

What season(s) am I experiencing?

Seasonal self-care

Thursday   Date   Moon phase ◯ Cycle day

How am I feeling?

What season(s) am I experiencing?

Seasonal self-care

You beautiful human, you are so precious.

Friday

Date .... Moon phase ◯ Cycle day ....

How am I feeling? ....

What season(s) am I experiencing? ....

Seasonal self-care ....

....

....

Saturday

Date .... Moon phase ◯ Cycle day ....

How am I feeling? ....

What season(s) am I experiencing? ....

Seasonal self-care ....

....

....

Sunday

Date .... Moon phase ◯ Cycle day ....

How am I feeling? ....

What season(s) am I experiencing? ....

Seasonal self-care ....

....

....

Weekly reflections

What's new?

What can I let go of?

Cycle Ten

MONTHLY REFLECTIONS

Another four weeks have passed, and you're poised on the brink of a new cycle. Though it might feel like a messy blur to you now, there is so much gold to be found in reflecting on your experiences. Wrap yourself in a blanket of self-love, have a flip through your journal pages from the previous weeks, check in with the Setting Intentions and Reflecting section in How to Use This Journal, and ponder the enquiries below.

What am I really proud of achieving?

Looking back at the last few months' moon charts, what patterns are occurring?

What new things are emerging for me?

What can I let go of?

What intentions can I make for next month?

MOON CHART

Date of new moon...

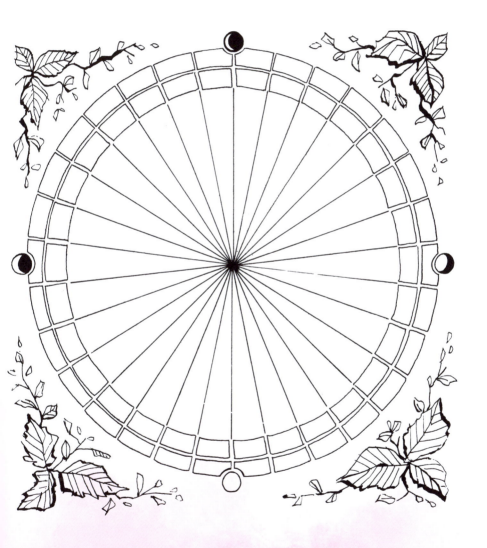

Monday   Date   Moon phase ◯   Cycle day

How am I feeling?

What season(s) am I experiencing?

Seasonal self-care

Tuesday   Date   Moon phase ◯   Cycle day

How am I feeling?

What season(s) am I experiencing?

Seasonal self-care

Wednesday   Date   Moon phase ◯   Cycle day

How am I feeling?

What season(s) am I experiencing?

Seasonal self-care

Thursday   Date   Moon phase ◯   Cycle day

How am I feeling?

What season(s) am I experiencing?

Seasonal self-care

The world desperately needs you and your special gifts.

Friday
Date .... Moon phase ◯ Cycle day ....

How am I feeling? ....

What season(s) am I experiencing? ....

Seasonal self-care ....

....

....

Saturday
Date .... Moon phase ◯ Cycle day ....

How am I feeling? ....

What season(s) am I experiencing? ....

Seasonal self-care ....

....

....

Sunday
Date .... Moon phase ◯ Cycle day ....

How am I feeling? ....

What season(s) am I experiencing? ....

Seasonal self-care ....

....

....

Weekly reflections

What's new?

What can I let go of?

Monday Date _____   Moon phase ◯ Cycle day _____

How am I feeling? _____

What season(s) am I experiencing? _____

Seasonal self-care _____

_____

_____

Tuesday Date _____   Moon phase ◯ Cycle day _____

How am I feeling? _____

What season(s) am I experiencing? _____

Seasonal self-care _____

_____

_____

Wednesday Date _____   Moon phase ◯ Cycle day _____

How am I feeling? _____

What season(s) am I experiencing? _____

Seasonal self-care _____

_____

_____

Thursday Date _____   Moon phase ◯ Cycle day _____

How am I feeling? _____

What season(s) am I experiencing? _____

Seasonal self-care _____

_____

_____

Look to nature for the deep wisdom of the seasons.

Friday   Date _____   Moon phase ◯ Cycle day _____

How am I feeling? _____

What season(s) am I experiencing? _____

Seasonal self-care _____

_____

Saturday   Date _____   Moon phase ◯ Cycle day _____

How am I feeling? _____

What season(s) am I experiencing? _____

Seasonal self-care _____

_____

Sunday   Date _____   Moon phase ◯ Cycle day _____

How am I feeling? _____

What season(s) am I experiencing? _____

Seasonal self-care _____

_____

Weekly reflections

What's new?

What can I let go of?

Monday   Date ....   Moon phase ◯ Cycle day ....

How am I feeling? ....

What season(s) am I experiencing? ....

Seasonal self-care ....

....

....

Tuesday   Date ....   Moon phase ◯ Cycle day ....

How am I feeling? ....

What season(s) am I experiencing? ....

Seasonal self-care ....

....

....

Wednesday Date ....   Moon phase ◯ Cycle day ....

How am I feeling? ....

What season(s) am I experiencing? ....

Seasonal self-care ....

....

....

Thursday   Date ....   Moon phase ◯ Cycle day ....

How am I feeling? ....

What season(s) am I experiencing? ....

Seasonal self-care ....

....

....

Only you know if a treatment is working: you're the expert on you.

Friday

Date .... Moon phase ◯ Cycle day ....

How am I feeling? ....

What season(s) am I experiencing? ....

Seasonal self-care ....

....

Saturday

Date .... Moon phase ◯ Cycle day ....

How am I feeling? ....

What season(s) am I experiencing? ....

Seasonal self-care ....

....

Sunday

Date .... Moon phase ◯ Cycle day ....

How am I feeling? ....

What season(s) am I experiencing? ....

Seasonal self-care ....

....

Weekly reflections

What's new?

What can I let go of?

Monday   Date   Moon phase ◯ Cycle day

How am I feeling?

What season(s) am I experiencing?

Seasonal self-care

_____

_____

Tuesday   Date   Moon phase ◯ Cycle day

How am I feeling?

What season(s) am I experiencing?

Seasonal self-care

_____

_____

Wednesday   Date   Moon phase ◯ Cycle day

How am I feeling?

What season(s) am I experiencing?

Seasonal self-care

_____

_____

Thursday   Date   Moon phase ◯ Cycle day

How am I feeling?

What season(s) am I experiencing?

Seasonal self-care

_____

_____

Lean in to the people who get you, lean away those who don't.

Friday   Date .... Moon phase ◯ Cycle day ....

How am I feeling? ....

What season(s) am I experiencing? ....

Seasonal self-care ....

....

Saturday   Date .... Moon phase ◯ Cycle day ....

How am I feeling? ....

What season(s) am I experiencing? ....

Seasonal self-care ....

....

Sunday   Date .... Moon phase ◯ Cycle day ....

How am I feeling? ....

What season(s) am I experiencing? ....

Seasonal self-care ....

....

Weekly reflections

What's new?

What can I let go of?

Cycle Eleven

MONTHLY REFLECTIONS

Another four weeks have passed, and you're poised on the brink of a new cycle. Though it might feel like a messy blur to you now, there is so much gold to be found in reflecting on your experiences. Wrap yourself in a blanket of self-love, have a flip through your journal pages from the previous weeks, check in with the Setting Intentions and Reflecting section in How to Use This Journal, and ponder the enquiries below.

What am I really proud of achieving?

Looking back at the last few months' moon charts, what patterns are occurring?

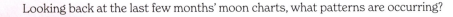

What new things are emerging for me?

What can I let go of?

What intentions can I make for next month?

MOON CHART

Date of new moon...

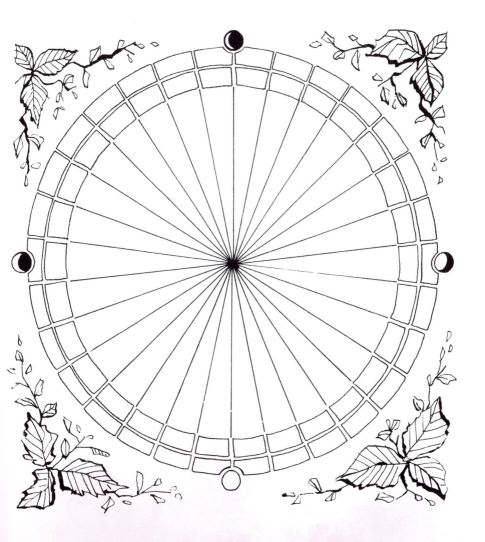

Monday   Date _____   Moon phase ◯ Cycle day _____

How am I feeling? _____

What season(s) am I experiencing? _____

Seasonal self-care _____

_____

_____

Tuesday   Date _____   Moon phase ◯ Cycle day _____

How am I feeling? _____

What season(s) am I experiencing? _____

Seasonal self-care _____

_____

_____

Wednesday   Date _____   Moon phase ◯ Cycle day _____

How am I feeling? _____

What season(s) am I experiencing? _____

Seasonal self-care _____

_____

_____

Thursday   Date _____   Moon phase ◯ Cycle day _____

How am I feeling? _____

What season(s) am I experiencing? _____

Seasonal self-care _____

_____

_____

Abandon controlling, embrace unfurling.

Friday
Date .... Moon phase ⃝ Cycle day ....

How am I feeling? ....

What season(s) am I experiencing? ....

Seasonal self-care ....

....

Saturday
Date .... Moon phase ⃝ Cycle day ....

How am I feeling? ....

What season(s) am I experiencing? ....

Seasonal self-care ....

....

Sunday
Date .... Moon phase ⃝ Cycle day ....

How am I feeling? ....

What season(s) am I experiencing? ....

Seasonal self-care ....

....

Weekly reflections

What's new?

What can I let go of?

Monday   Date ....   Moon phase ◯   Cycle day ....

How am I feeling? ....

What season(s) am I experiencing? ....

Seasonal self-care ....

....

....

Tuesday   Date ....   Moon phase ◯   Cycle day ....

How am I feeling? ....

What season(s) am I experiencing? ....

Seasonal self-care ....

....

....

Wednesday   Date ....   Moon phase ◯   Cycle day ....

How am I feeling? ....

What season(s) am I experiencing? ....

Seasonal self-care ....

....

....

Thursday   Date ....   Moon phase ◯   Cycle day ....

How am I feeling? ....

What season(s) am I experiencing? ....

Seasonal self-care ....

....

....

It's time to remove the armour of fear and allow yourself to be seen for the glorious human you are.

Friday

Date .... Moon phase ◯ Cycle day ....

How am I feeling? ....

What season(s) am I experiencing? ....

Seasonal self-care ....

....

Saturday

Date .... Moon phase ◯ Cycle day ....

How am I feeling? ....

What season(s) am I experiencing? ....

Seasonal self-care ....

....

Sunday

Date .... Moon phase ◯ Cycle day ....

How am I feeling? ....

What season(s) am I experiencing? ....

Seasonal self-care ....

....

Weekly reflections

What's new?

What can I let go of?

Monday   Date   Moon phase ◯ Cycle day

How am I feeling?

What season(s) am I experiencing?

Seasonal self-care

Tuesday   Date   Moon phase ◯ Cycle day

How am I feeling?

What season(s) am I experiencing?

Seasonal self-care

Wednesday   Date   Moon phase ◯ Cycle day

How am I feeling?

What season(s) am I experiencing?

Seasonal self-care

Thursday   Date   Moon phase ◯ Cycle day

How am I feeling?

What season(s) am I experiencing?

Seasonal self-care

Everything is not just 'ok' — everything is waking up!

Friday
Date .... Moon phase ◯ Cycle day ....
How am I feeling? ....
What season(s) am I experiencing? ....
Seasonal self-care ....

Saturday
Date .... Moon phase ◯ Cycle day ....
How am I feeling? ....
What season(s) am I experiencing? ....
Seasonal self-care ....

Sunday
Date .... Moon phase ◯ Cycle day ....
How am I feeling? ....
What season(s) am I experiencing? ....
Seasonal self-care ....

Weekly reflections

What's new?

What can I let go of?

Monday   Date............................   Moon phase ◯   Cycle day............

How am I feeling?...

What season(s) am I experiencing?...

Seasonal self-care...

....

....

Tuesday   Date............................   Moon phase ◯   Cycle day............

How am I feeling?...

What season(s) am I experiencing?...

Seasonal self-care...

....

....

Wednesday   Date............................   Moon phase ◯   Cycle day............

How am I feeling?...

What season(s) am I experiencing?...

Seasonal self-care...

....

....

Thursday   Date............................   Moon phase ◯   Cycle day............

How am I feeling?...

What season(s) am I experiencing?...

Seasonal self-care...

....

....

Perimenopause is your soul breaking free of your conditioning.

Friday
Date _____ Moon phase ◯ Cycle day _____

How am I feeling? _____

What season(s) am I experiencing? _____

Seasonal self-care _____

_____

_____

Saturday
Date _____ Moon phase ◯ Cycle day _____

How am I feeling? _____

What season(s) am I experiencing? _____

Seasonal self-care _____

_____

_____

Sunday
Date _____ Moon phase ◯ Cycle day _____

How am I feeling? _____

What season(s) am I experiencing? _____

Seasonal self-care _____

_____

_____

Weekly reflections

What's new?

What can I let go of?

Cycle Twelve

MONTHLY REFLECTIONS

Another four weeks have passed, and you're poised on the brink of a new cycle. Though it might feel like a messy blur to you now, there is so much gold to be found in reflecting on your experiences. Wrap yourself in a blanket of self-love, have a flip through your journal pages from the previous weeks, check in with the Setting Intentions and Reflecting section in How to Use This Journal, and ponder the enquiries below.

What am I really proud of achieving?

Looking back at the last few months' moon charts, what patterns are occurring?

What new things are emerging for me?

What can I let go of?

What intentions can I make for next month?

MOON CHART

Date of new moon...

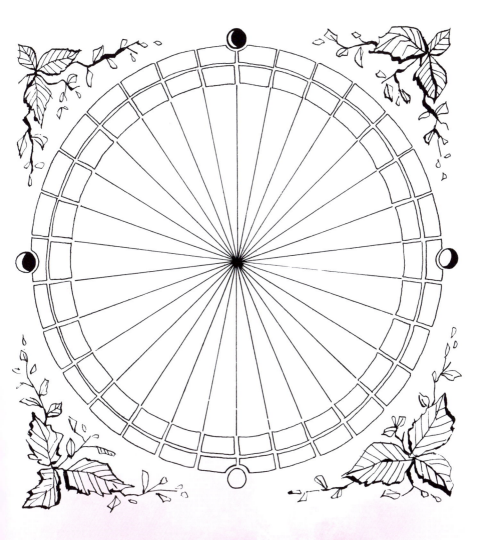

Monday   Date ....   Moon phase ◯   Cycle day ....

How am I feeling? ....

What season(s) am I experiencing? ....

Seasonal self-care ....

....

....

Tuesday   Date ....   Moon phase ◯   Cycle day ....

How am I feeling? ....

What season(s) am I experiencing? ....

Seasonal self-care ....

....

....

Wednesday   Date ....   Moon phase ◯   Cycle day ....

How am I feeling? ....

What season(s) am I experiencing? ....

Seasonal self-care ....

....

....

Thursday   Date ....   Moon phase ◯   Cycle day ....

How am I feeling? ....

What season(s) am I experiencing? ....

Seasonal self-care ....

....

....

Autumn is the time to embody your wisdom. Be bold!

Friday
Date .... Moon phase ◯ Cycle day ....

How am I feeling? ....

What season(s) am I experiencing? ....

Seasonal self-care ....

....

....

Saturday
Date .... Moon phase ◯ Cycle day ....

How am I feeling? ....

What season(s) am I experiencing? ....

Seasonal self-care ....

....

....

Sunday
Date .... Moon phase ◯ Cycle day ....

How am I feeling? ....

What season(s) am I experiencing? ....

Seasonal self-care ....

....

....

Weekly reflections

What's new?

What can I let go of?

Monday   Date ....   Moon phase ◯ Cycle day ....

How am I feeling? ....

What season(s) am I experiencing? ....

Seasonal self-care ....

....

....

Tuesday   Date ....   Moon phase ◯ Cycle day ....

How am I feeling? ....

What season(s) am I experiencing? ....

Seasonal self-care ....

....

....

Wednesday Date ....   Moon phase ◯ Cycle day ....

How am I feeling? ....

What season(s) am I experiencing? ....

Seasonal self-care ....

....

....

Thursday   Date ....   Moon phase ◯ Cycle day ....

How am I feeling? ....

What season(s) am I experiencing? ....

Seasonal self-care ....

....

....

Take refuge in the senses: delight in colour, texture, taste, smell and sound.

Friday
Date _____ Moon phase ◯ Cycle day _____

How am I feeling? _____

What season(s) am I experiencing? _____

Seasonal self-care _____

_____

Saturday
Date _____ Moon phase ◯ Cycle day _____

How am I feeling? _____

What season(s) am I experiencing? _____

Seasonal self-care _____

_____

Sunday
Date _____ Moon phase ◯ Cycle day _____

How am I feeling? _____

What season(s) am I experiencing? _____

Seasonal self-care _____

_____

Weekly reflections

What's new?

What can I let go of?

Monday   Date _____   Moon phase ○ Cycle day _____

How am I feeling? _____

What season(s) am I experiencing? _____

Seasonal self-care _____

_____

_____

Tuesday   Date _____   Moon phase ○ Cycle day _____

How am I feeling? _____

What season(s) am I experiencing? _____

Seasonal self-care _____

_____

_____

Wednesday   Date _____   Moon phase ○ Cycle day _____

How am I feeling? _____

What season(s) am I experiencing? _____

Seasonal self-care _____

_____

_____

Thursday   Date _____   Moon phase ○ Cycle day _____

How am I feeling? _____

What season(s) am I experiencing? _____

Seasonal self-care _____

_____

_____

Feeling angry? How might you channel this energy for good?

Friday

Date .... Moon phase ◯ Cycle day ....

How am I feeling? ....

What season(s) am I experiencing? ....

Seasonal self-care ....

....

....

Saturday

Date .... Moon phase ◯ Cycle day ....

How am I feeling? ....

What season(s) am I experiencing? ....

Seasonal self-care ....

....

....

Sunday

Date .... Moon phase ◯ Cycle day ....

How am I feeling? ....

What season(s) am I experiencing? ....

Seasonal self-care ....

....

....

Weekly reflections

What's new?

What can I let go of?

Monday   Date ....   Moon phase ◯   Cycle day ....

How am I feeling? ....

What season(s) am I experiencing? ....

Seasonal self-care ....

....

....

Tuesday   Date ....   Moon phase ◯   Cycle day ....

How am I feeling? ....

What season(s) am I experiencing? ....

Seasonal self-care ....

....

....

Wednesday   Date ....   Moon phase ◯   Cycle day ....

How am I feeling? ....

What season(s) am I experiencing? ....

Seasonal self-care ....

....

....

Thursday   Date ....   Moon phase ◯   Cycle day ....

How am I feeling? ....

What season(s) am I experiencing? ....

Seasonal self-care ....

....

....

Swap 'selfish' for being more self-ish!

Friday
Date .... Moon phase ○ Cycle day ....

How am I feeling? ....

What season(s) am I experiencing? ....

Seasonal self-care ....

....

Saturday
Date .... Moon phase ○ Cycle day ....

How am I feeling? ....

What season(s) am I experiencing? ....

Seasonal self-care ....

....

Sunday
Date .... Moon phase ○ Cycle day ....

How am I feeling? ....

What season(s) am I experiencing? ....

Seasonal self-care ....

....

Weekly reflections

What's new?

What can I let go of?

Cycle Thirteen

MONTHLY REFLECTIONS

Another four weeks have passed, and you're poised on the brink of a new cycle. Though it might feel like a messy blur to you now, there is so much gold to be found in reflecting on your experiences. Wrap yourself in a blanket of self-love, have a flip through your journal pages from the previous weeks, check in with the Setting Intentions and Reflecting section in How to Use This Journal, and ponder the enquiries below.

What am I really proud of achieving?

Looking back at the last few months' moon charts, what patterns are occurring?

What new things are emerging for me?

What can I let go of?

What intentions can I make for next month?

MOON CHART

Date of new moon...

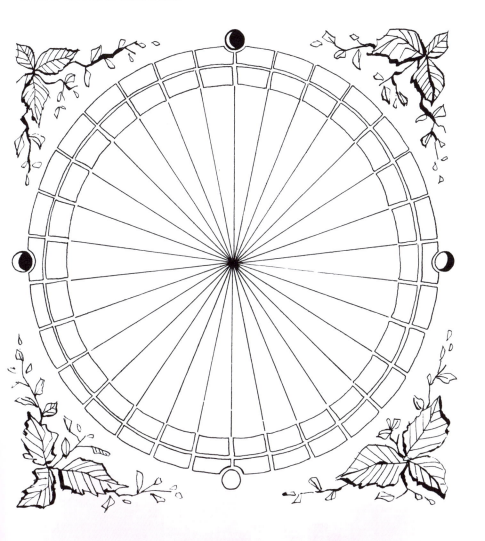

Monday   Date ....   Moon phase ◯   Cycle day ....

How am I feeling? ....

What season(s) am I experiencing? ....

Seasonal self-care ....

....

....

Tuesday   Date ....   Moon phase ◯   Cycle day ....

How am I feeling? ....

What season(s) am I experiencing? ....

Seasonal self-care ....

....

....

Wednesday   Date ....   Moon phase ◯   Cycle day ....

How am I feeling? ....

What season(s) am I experiencing? ....

Seasonal self-care ....

....

....

Thursday   Date ....   Moon phase ◯   Cycle day ....

How am I feeling? ....

What season(s) am I experiencing? ....

Seasonal self-care ....

....

....

Be your own best friend and love the hell out of yourself.

Friday   Date _____   Moon phase ◯ Cycle day _____

How am I feeling? _____

What season(s) am I experiencing? _____

Seasonal self-care _____

_____

Saturday   Date _____   Moon phase ◯ Cycle day _____

How am I feeling? _____

What season(s) am I experiencing? _____

Seasonal self-care _____

_____

Sunday   Date _____   Moon phase ◯ Cycle day _____

How am I feeling? _____

What season(s) am I experiencing? _____

Seasonal self-care _____

_____

Weekly reflections

What's new?

What can I let go of?

Monday   Date ....   Moon phase ◯ Cycle day ....

How am I feeling? ....

What season(s) am I experiencing? ....

Seasonal self-care ....

....

....

Tuesday   Date ....   Moon phase ◯ Cycle day ....

How am I feeling? ....

What season(s) am I experiencing? ....

Seasonal self-care ....

....

....

Wednesday   Date ....   Moon phase ◯ Cycle day ....

How am I feeling? ....

What season(s) am I experiencing? ....

Seasonal self-care ....

....

....

Thursday   Date ....   Moon phase ◯ Cycle day ....

How am I feeling? ....

What season(s) am I experiencing? ....

Seasonal self-care ....

....

....

How could you safely express your feelings in this moment?

Friday

Date _____ Moon phase ◯ Cycle day _____

How am I feeling? _____

What season(s) am I experiencing? _____

Seasonal self-care _____

_____

Saturday

Date _____ Moon phase ◯ Cycle day _____

How am I feeling? _____

What season(s) am I experiencing? _____

Seasonal self-care _____

_____

Sunday

Date _____ Moon phase ◯ Cycle day _____

How am I feeling? _____

What season(s) am I experiencing? _____

Seasonal self-care _____

_____

Weekly reflections

What's new?

What can I let go of?

Monday   Date _____   Moon phase ◯   Cycle day _____

How am I feeling? _____

What season(s) am I experiencing? _____

Seasonal self-care _____

_____

_____

Tuesday   Date _____   Moon phase ◯   Cycle day _____

How am I feeling? _____

What season(s) am I experiencing? _____

Seasonal self-care _____

_____

_____

Wednesday   Date _____   Moon phase ◯   Cycle day _____

How am I feeling? _____

What season(s) am I experiencing? _____

Seasonal self-care _____

_____

_____

Thursday   Date _____   Moon phase ◯   Cycle day _____

How am I feeling? _____

What season(s) am I experiencing? _____

Seasonal self-care _____

_____

_____

Suffering shows you there's something wrong for you, not with you.

Friday   Date   Moon phase ◯ Cycle day

How am I feeling?

What season(s) am I experiencing?

Seasonal self-care

Saturday   Date   Moon phase ◯ Cycle day

How am I feeling?

What season(s) am I experiencing?

Seasonal self-care

Sunday   Date   Moon phase ◯ Cycle day

How am I feeling?

What season(s) am I experiencing?

Seasonal self-care

Weekly reflections

What's new?

What can I let go of?

Monday　　Date _____　　Moon phase ◯　　Cycle day _____

How am I feeling? ....

What season(s) am I experiencing? ....

Seasonal self-care ....

....

Tuesday　　Date _____　　Moon phase ◯　　Cycle day _____

How am I feeling? ....

What season(s) am I experiencing? ....

Seasonal self-care ....

....

Wednesday　　Date _____　　Moon phase ◯　　Cycle day _____

How am I feeling? ....

What season(s) am I experiencing? ....

Seasonal self-care ....

....

Thursday　　Date _____　　Moon phase ◯　　Cycle day _____

How am I feeling? ....

What season(s) am I experiencing? ....

Seasonal self-care ....

....

Stepping away from what is not serving you is an act of care.

Friday
Date .... Moon phase ◯ Cycle day

How am I feeling? ....

What season(s) am I experiencing? ....

Seasonal self-care ....

....

....

Saturday
Date .... Moon phase ◯ Cycle day

How am I feeling? ....

What season(s) am I experiencing? ....

Seasonal self-care ....

....

....

Sunday
Date .... Moon phase ◯ Cycle day

How am I feeling? ....

What season(s) am I experiencing? ....

Seasonal self-care ....

....

....

Weekly reflections

What's new?

What can I let go of?

Some Final Reflections...

You are amazing. Just by witnessing your feelings and showing up to care for yourself, you've evolved into a whole new mindset. Take a few moments to flip through your journal and appreciate all that you've done for yourself, then answer these prompts to reflect on your year of caring for yourself:

- What has energised me?

- What has drained me?

- What was I required to let go of?

- What was I asked to accept?

- What am I most grateful for?

- What am I most proud of?

- How have I grown?

- How can I care for myself better next year?

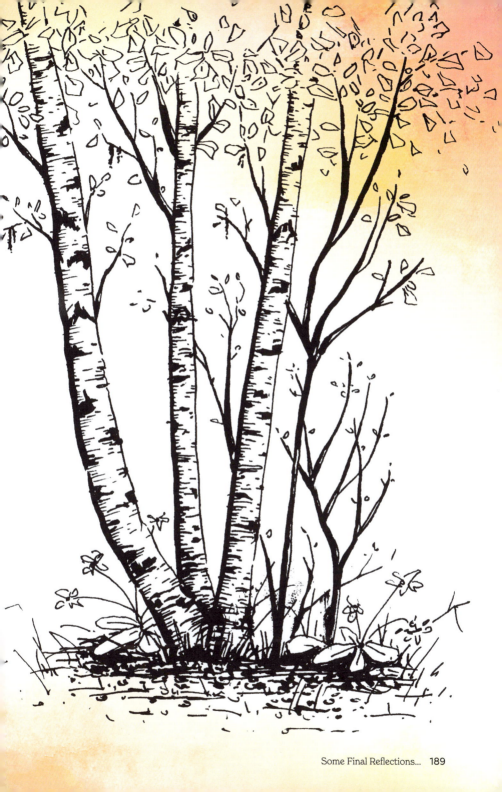

Thoughts For Your Journey...

I'm just dropping in here to remind you that you are amazing; a unique, beautiful human shining your own particular light in your own particular way. A year has passed since you started tracking your inner seasons and noticing how you might care for yourself. Doubtless your inner critic will be biting your heels and saying you 'should have journalled more', or 'done more' or 'less' or 'better' or something – that's inevitable. But coming back into relationship with ourselves is neither simple nor linear. If it was, we'd have done it years ago! If you had been taught at home and school how to balance your needs and serve the world authentically with your unique gifts, you wouldn't be here trying to figure it out now. I've said it a few times, but it's worth repeating: just the act of paying mindful attention to the ebbs and flow of the seasons is more than enough.

Paying gentle attention to your seasons makes every day meaningful. So often we plod along in the hope of arriving 'elsewhere' where the grass is greener and we are happier, more successful humans, but this takes our attention away from the magic right under our nose. Each day the seasons show up some part of ourselves that is asking to be integrated. Perhaps the child who believed in fairies, the honouring of an ancestral persecution, or the burning flame of rage against injustice. The seasons show us that this process of integration is present bubbling away just beneath our everyday struggles, helping us reclaim what we have lost. Bringing loving care to your seasons through the sensitive perimenopause years is setting you up for your second half of life.

Not that it's comfortable though – perimenopause is a revolution! It shakes us up into a hot mess so we question which way is up, and this is necessary. It's from this messy, confused space we can let go of what's not serving us and kick it in the bum. Be it relationships, friendships, toxic habits, eating patterns or chronic over-giving, it's time to change and start to treat yourself with the dignity and respect you deserve. For yourself yes, but also so you can bring your own gifts and skills into the world in a sustainable way, and serve your community. If you can't do it for yourself, if it feels too selfish or narcissistic to give the time to nourish yourself, do it to be a good role model. After all, if you continue to the point of burnout, what is that teaching your co-workers, friends and the younger generation?

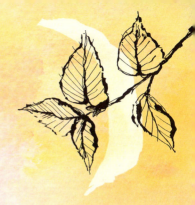

I know it might feel like it goes on forever, but perimenopause is a transition where you are sensitive and need care. It is often mistaken for the beginnings of the slippery slope of decrepitude, but this is not the case: once your hormones level out you enter the 'kinder and gentler life-phase' of postmenopause as endocrinologist Dr Jerilynn Prior calls it. Human happiness is U-shaped, dipping for everyone in your 40s and 50s and then on an upwards trajectory from your mid-50s onwards. Postmenopausal life, from your Second Spring onwards, brings a calmness, joy and clarity that was missing in earlier years.

Having one remaining member of the older generation in my family, sprightly and shiny-eyed as she is, I find that my sisters and I have now been shunted into the 'old dears' spot at family gatherings. How did this happen? We're still feeling like teens inside! Soon there will be no old-timer wisdom to lean into and we will be the elders. As I travel further into my second cycle of life, I notice an increasing longing for role models and teachers, for women in their 70s and 80s who are uncompromisingly themselves. Who shine with delight at being alive, and utilise their abundant curiosity and compassion to connect deeply with those around them. We need these people to show us the way, and ultimately we need to become these people.

We need a generation of strong, healthy postmenopausal folk like you to help us get out of the mess we're in. You may be the person who feeds the birds or runs a business empire, has that heart-lifting smile or stands on top of the barricades – any and all ways of being authentically yourself in a sustainable way will make a difference.

So wherever you are in your perimenopause journey, just showing up as yourself is the best possible gift you can give to the world, and we love you for it.

Go gently with your dear self.

Kate x

Further Reading & Resources

It's been a deliberate choice in this journal to support your unique experience and show you how you can use your perimenopause to integrate and become more wholly yourself. To dive more into symptoms, conditions, treatments, what to eat, how to move, HRT, supplements etc., here are some excellent resources.

Second Spring: The self-care guide to menopause by Kate Codrington – the low-down on all aspects of self-care with a seasonal frame.

Hormone Repair Manual by Lara Briden – clear explanation of hormones, conditions and treatments with nutrition, bioidentical hormones and supplements.

The Complete Guide to the Menopause by Annice Mukhurjee – comprehensive guide with great section on hormone therapy.

The Complete Guide to Breast Cancer by Professor Trisha Greenhalgh and Dr Liz O'Riordan – authors have both professional and personal experience of cancer. Thorough, compassionate, evidence-based.

Wise Power by Alexandra Pope and Sjanie Hugo Wurlitzer – inspirational dive into the transformational power of menopause.

Grow Your Own HRT by Sally J. Duffell – the science and practicalities of growing sprouts to manage hormone fluctuations.

Rebel Bodies: A guide to the gender health gap revolution by Sarah Graham – includes excellent section on how to advocate to get the diagnosis and treatment you need.

Moon Wise: How to find peace and power with the cycle of the moon by Awen Clement – guide to living in the rhythm of the moon and annual seasons.

Me And My Menopausal Vagina by Jane Lewis – warm, funny, informative guide to treating vaginal atrophy.

The Natural Menopause Method by Karen Newby – guide to using nutrition to manage symptoms.

What Fresh Hell is This? Perimenopause, menopause, other indignities and you by Heather Corinna – thoroughly inclusive, feminist guide to perimenopause.

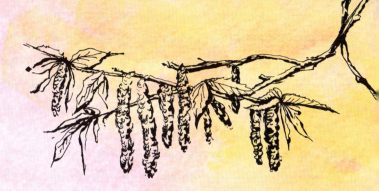

Magnificent Midlife: Transform your middle years, menopause and beyond by Rachel Lankester - radical, research-based rebranding of midlife and menopause.

Yoga Nidra Made Easy by Uma Dinsmore-Tuli and Nirlipta Tuli – empowering, practical beginner's guide to creating your own yoga nidra.

How to Break Up with Your Phone by Catherine Price - 30-day plan to get your life back.

The XX Brain by Dr Lisa Mosconi – female brains and preventing dementia.

Wild Feminine: Finding power, spirit and joy in the female body by Tami Lynn Kent – stuffed with practices and enquiries to heal and recover your best self.

Menopausal Years The Wise Woman Way by Susun S. Weed – the bible on herbs for menopause.

Organisations

The Eve Appeal for gynaecological health – resources and excellent helpline

Daisy Network – menopause before 40

HysterSisters - for those who have had or are considering hysterectomy

Breast Cancer UK – resources and information with comprehensive section on xenoestrogens

The Society for Women's Health Research - advancing women's health through science, policy, and education

NICE – UK guidelines for health and care with up-to-date perimenopause guide

International Association for Premenstrual Disorders or IAPMD - resources for women and AFAB individuals with Premenstrual Dysphoric Disorder (PMDD) and Premenstrual Exacerbation (PME)

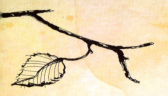

About the author

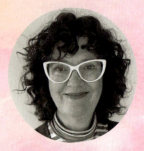

Kate is a writer, mentor, facilitator, yoga nidra guide, podcaster and artist. Her first book, *Second Spring: The self-care guide to menopause*, was hailed as one of the 'menopause cannon' by the *New York Times*. She has been a therapist for more than 30 years and lives in Watford with her partner and two adult children.

Acknowledgements

This book is dedicated to my beloved clients: if they knew how much I learn from their wisdom, persistence and self-love, I'd risk never getting paid again. I've taken inspiration from all the perimenopause warriors I have been lucky enough to come into contact with: clients, friends and colleagues who let their preciousness shine through, despite navigating the tricky waters of transformation, picking themselves up and dusting themselves down again and again to shine their beautiful light in the world. Lucky us!

The structure of the seasons is gifted by Alexandra Pope and Sjanie Hugo Wurlitzer of Red School, and I would never have reached this point of clarity without the love, sharp eye and fine mind of our dear Leora Leboff.

The Perimenopause Journal has been magicked from a daydream into the beautiful creation you are holding now, by hard work from a team of dedicated, creative good eggs who have stepped up to support it. I am indebted to Jane Graham Maw and her team at Graham Maw Christie, Lizzie Kaye and the editors and designers at David and Charles, Pru Rogers for her evocative, vibrant illustrations, not to mention the folk at the paper mills, ink makers, typesetters, printers, delivery drivers, retail staff, sales, PR and marketing teams, and many others who have made this beauty possible. I've only met a few of you, but thank you all!

Finally a thank you to my dear partner Ian, and the fine adults who were only recently known as 'my kids', for putting up with my shenanigans and generously allowing me the spaciousness needed to do my thing.

Index

A catalogue record for this book is available
from the British Library.

ISBN-13: 9781446313589 hardback

This book has been printed on paper from
approved suppliers and made from pulp from
sustainable sources.

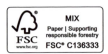

Printed in China through Asia Pacific Offset for:
David and Charles, Ltd, Suite A, Tourism House,
Pynes Hill, Exeter, EX2 5WS

10 9 8 7 6 5 4 3 2 1

Publishing Director: Ame Verso
Senior Commissioning Editor: Lizzie Kaye
Managing Editor: Jeni Chown
Editor: Victoria Allen
Project Editor: Jane Trollope
Head of Design: Anna Wade
Designers: Anna Wade & Jess Pearson
Pre-press Designer: Susan Reansbury
Illustrations: Pru Rogers
Production Manager: Beverley Richardson

David and Charles publishes high-quality
books on a wide range of subjects. For more
information visit www.davidandcharles.com

Follow us on Instagram by searching for
@dandcbooks_wellbeing.